MINIMALIST LIVING

Minimalist Living Principles for a Simpler Existence

(Brilliant Minimalism Tips to Declutter and Organize Your Home)

Charles Sabb

Published by Tomas Edwards

© **Charles Sabb**

All Rights Reserved

Minimalism Living: Minimalist Living Principles for a Simpler Existence (Brilliant Minimalism Tips to Declutter and Organize Your Home)

ISBN 978-1-989744-64-2

All rights reserved. No part of this guide may be reproduced in any form without permission in writing from the publisher except in the case of brief quotations embodied in critical articles or reviews.

Legal & Disclaimer

The information contained in this book is not designed to replace or take the place of any form of medicine or professional medical advice. The information in this book has been provided for educational and entertainment purposes only.

The information contained in this book has been compiled from sources deemed reliable, and it is accurate to the best of the Author's knowledge; however, the Author cannot guarantee its accuracy and validity and cannot be held liable for any errors or omissions. Changes are periodically made to this book. You must consult your doctor or get professional medical advice before using any of the suggested remedies, techniques, or information in this book.

Upon using the information contained in this book, you agree to hold harmless the Author from and against any damages, costs, and expenses, including any legal fees potentially resulting from the application of any of the information provided by this guide. This disclaimer applies to any damages or injury caused by the use and application, whether directly or indirectly, of any advice or information presented, whether for breach of contract, tort, negligence, personal injury, criminal intent, or under any other cause of action.

You agree to accept all risks of using the information presented inside this book. You need to consult a professional medical practitioner in order to ensure you are both able and healthy enough to participate in this program.

Table of Contents

INTRODUCTION 1

CHAPTER 1: GET FOCUSED 3

CHAPTER 2: PERKS OF MINIMALISM AND DECLUTTERING, ACCORDING TO SCIENCE 16

CHAPTER 3: THE HOARDING CRISIS - WHY MODERN SOCIETY IS FOCUSED ON ACCUMULATING MATERIAL POSSESSIONS 24

CHAPTER 4: DECLUTTER 33

CHAPTER 5: THE PROMISES OF CONSUMERISM 46

CHAPTER 6: LESSENING THE CLUTTER............................. 59

CHAPTER 7: THE INITIAL STEPS TO A MINIMALISTIC WAY OF LIFE 65

CHAPTER 8: THE TRANSITION 74

CHAPTER 9: THE PROCESS OF DECLUTTERING 87

CHAPTER 10: THE BENEFITS OF MINIMALISM................. 94

CHAPTER 11: 7 STEP SYSTEM TO MINIMALISM AND DECLUTTERING ANYTHING 113

CHAPTER 12: POSSESSIONS: LESS IS MORE.................... 127

CHAPTER 13: BY CHOOSING TO BE A MINIMALIST, YOU WILL BE MORE PRODUCTIVE 142

CHAPTER 14: EXPERIENCING LIFE MORE MEANS OVERCOMING CONVENIENCE ADDICTION.................... 151

CHAPTER 15: WAYS YOU CAN EMBRACE MINIMALISM EVERY DAY 159

CHAPTER 16: MINIMALISM AND DISCIPLINE 164

CHAPTER 17: MINIMALIST WARDROBE 172

CHAPTER 18: EXPLORING MINIMALISM AND HEALTH ... 180

CHAPTER 19: DECLUTTER THE LIVING ROOM................. 185

CHAPTER 20: DECLUTTER YOUR DIGITAL LIFE 195

CONCLUSION... 201

Introduction

Minimalism helps you appreciate non material things such as experiences and skills. Experiences are much more enriching than material possessions and aren't as expensive most of the time. Yes, traveling might be an expensive activity but you come back with stories to tell your family and friends about how snorkelling changed your perception of the sea or how the daily morning hike made you realise how lucky you are or that incredible restaurant in which you tried the freshest fish you've ever had or that you had access to the tastiest, sweetest fruit every single morning for breakfast. Plus, you don't have to travel with more than a carry-on since everything you need fits there.

Once you start downsizing it becomes rather addictive, you find yourself with more time and energy to do whatever it is you truly enjoy doing. It is liberating.

Freedom at it's truest form. Once you own less you learn to appreciate every single one of your items for the purpose it fulfils or the utility it has.

In today's world where it is all about acquiring fancy new things, it is hard to imagine that having less could be beneficial to us. What could be bad about having nice, fancy cars in front of one of your biggest properties filled with all the latest gadgets and fine furniture? For some people, there may be nothing wrong with it but if you are reading this, you may have noticed that your material possessions have not brought you the happiness you were expecting. If this is the case you may be ready to get more from less. Again, I'm not hating on the luxury lifestyle. If you have enough to afford it and you want it, I'd say go for it but the problem becomes apparent when you can't afford to have those cars and properties and yet still hold on to them and they drag you further into debt.

Chapter 1: Get Focused

Before you ever embark on a new journey, it is important to get focused and clear on what you are doing. You want to know exactly why you are taking on a new journey or path, and what this lifestyle will mean for you. Getting focused gives you the opportunity to completely understand what your motives and intentions are and why you should stay committed when things get difficult, which they always do at one point or another.

With minimalism, you should understand that the lifestyle is more than just living a life free of physical clutter. It is also about living a life free of mental, emotional, and non-physical clutter. You need to learn to stay focused on what you want and stop dwelling on things that do not serve you and have no purpose in your life. You can do that by getting focused and staying clear on what your goals are.

Initially, getting focused might be extremely simple. There are usually two reasons why someone wants to become a minimalist: either they cannot stand looking around at clutter anymore, or they cannot stand all of the restrictions on their time. Because both of these involve stress and discomfort, people are driven to make a change in their life. However, it can be easy to stop making changes once you reach a place of comfort. Or, you may not want to begin because you realize that any change will be less comfortable than what you are already doing. After all, we tend to stay in lifestyles that are most comfortable to us.

It is important that you learn that staying focused and determined takes effort on a constant basis. Focus is a balancing act that you must work towards constantly. The more you work towards it, the more success you are going to have with it. The following tips are going to help you both with getting focused and clear on your path, and with learning to re-center your focus along the way. You will be guided through a couple of journaling exercises which will give you a great opportunity to get clear and give yourself something to refer back to when it gets difficult. These activities are important to your success, so it is a good idea to actually invest the time in completing them.

Tip #1: Write Down your Reasons

The very first step to getting clear is knowing exactly what your reasons are behind becoming a minimalist. You need to know what is compelling you to make the change, and why you are so dedicated. It is important that you are completely clear on why you are making these changes and that the reasons are important to you. When we are passionate about our purpose, we are much more likely to succeed in what we set out to accomplish.

While you are getting clear on your reasons, take out a piece of paper and write them down. Some people may benefit from simply writing this down on a page in their journal, whereas others may want to take some time with it and turn their reasons into a piece of art that they can keep in a highly visible spot each day. What you choose to do will be up to you, but the most important thing is that you have your reasons readily available.

When you embark on a new journey in life, it can be easy to have mental "relapses" which will draw you back into a previous way of thinking. You may fall back into old habits or patterns and think "well, just this once!" But it's that exact mindset that leads you towards having a cluttered environment. It is during times like this that you want to go back to your written list of reasons and feel into them. Feel the emotion you put behind them and let it rise to the surface for you. The more you can truly feel those emotions, the easier it will be for you to remember why you are a minimalist and stay true to your desires.

Tip #2: Reclaim Your Time

So much time is wasted when you are trapped in a lifestyle that is solely focused on acquiring the latest and greatest. You spend several hours working, often at a job you don't even like. This generates stress, grief, anger, frustration, and other unwanted emotions that you must face on a regular basis. Then, you must spend time maintaining all of the objects you have acquired. You need to organize them, reorganize them, clean them, service them, and otherwise maintain them. Then, you need to actually find the time to use them, which you likely rarely ever do find so you often end up acquiring objects that simply sit around for you to look at. If you travel or go anywhere you likely bring more than is required simply because you are too guilty to leave something behind knowing that you spent your precious money on it, which is a direct symbol for time in your subconscious and potentially even in your conscious mind. Then, of course, you must invest time in acquiring more. So, you spend several hours in stores and malls getting frustrated over lineups, other shoppers, and anything else that may upset you. You may go into debt to acquire new things, or you may simply scrape by paycheck to paycheck because you don't want to stop purchasing new belongings. It can be a difficult trap to get stuck in.

Being a minimalist means that you get to reclaim your time. You get to stop working so hard to earn money to pay for items you don't have time to use, much less properly maintain. You get to stop spending hours a day working to pay off debt, cleaning, and staring at your house full of unused objects. You get the chance to completely free yourself from all of the burdens that come along with these actions, both emotionally and physically. Ultimately, you get to reclaim your time to live a life that you want. You can do anything you want with the time that you reclaim, the choice is entirely up to you.

In the beginning, it is a great idea to take a page from your journal and write down all of the things you wish you had time for.

What do you want to do that you haven't done because you don't have time? What are the things that you have been putting off because there never seems to be a spare moment for you to complete them? How are you suffering in your own life because you don't give yourself enough time to enjoy it? This list is something you should refer to on a regular basis. As you adopt the minimalist lifestyle, you will want to start checking things off of this list. If you ever feel unsure of what to do or where to go next, use this list as an opportunity to guide you. You can even build on the list as new ideas come up, regardless of how far or deep into your minimalist journey.

The greatest part of being a minimalist is all of the free time you have. Many minimalists are even able to reduce their hours and go down to working part time instead of full time because they simply don't need all of the extra money and they would rather spend time enjoying their life. Many even get to quit their job altogether and pursue a career that they are passionate about because they are no longer fearful of what will happen if they don't have a job to return to should anything go wrong. The freedom that you gain from minimalism is unparalleled, and it is something you can look forward to enjoying in your own minimalist journey.

Tip #3: What Do You Value?

A major part of the minimalist journey is learning about what you value most. When you are clear on what matters most to you, then you know exactly how to spend your time and resources on creating a life that you love, which is what minimalism is all about. You should spend some time getting to know what you value and becoming clear on it.

A great way to do this is to take your journal and start journaling. Write down what matters most to you, and what you want to gain from life. What experiences make you feel rich with joy and happiness? What makes you excited to wake up and experience each new day as it comes? These are the things you want to enrich your life with. You should give yourself the opportunity to experience these as often as possible. When you are a minimalist, you have less to worry about in regards of taking care of your belongings and gaining more. Instead, you have the gift of more free time, which means that you get to spend your free time however you want.

The other reason why it is important to know what you value is because it allows you to decide what you want to purchase and own in life. For example, if you value the ability to hop in the car and go anywhere then you may want to keep your car, whereas if you don't mind taking public transit it may be more beneficial if you get rid of your car. The same goes for virtually anything else you may own.

Tip #4: Saying "No"

Learning to say "no" is important, and it should be one of the first things you learn as a minimalist. You need to know how to say no to bringing more belongings into your house, how to say no to keeping belongings in your house, and how to say no to doing things you don't want to do.

Many people believe minimalism is all about items, but it's not. It's about your time and your lifestyle as well. It is about eliminating anything that does not serve your highest good, and learning to say no to anything that does not bring you joy. You want to learn how to say no and mean it, and never waiver in your answer. There is never a good enough reason to do something that does not make you feel good overall.

Saying "no" can be hard at first, especially if you are really not used to doing it. The more you practice, however, the easier it will be. You should learn to say no to smaller things first: shopping, bringing things home, joining e-mail newsletters, and other easier things. As you get used to it and it becomes easier for you, you can start saying it to bigger things that may be harder for you: going out with people, getting rid of sentimental things that you do not value, and bringing things you like home when you know you won't use them much.

Tip #5: Minimalism is a Journey

Minimalism is a journey, not a linear goal. You are not going to wake up one morning with a trophy on your shelf because you 'accomplished' minimalism. Instead, minimalism is a lifestyle. You are going to be working towards your minimalist lifestyle for the rest of your life, or until you no longer desire to be a minimalist. But fear not, if you aren't already in love with it most people find that they do become passionate about minimalism and therefore it becomes easier to maintain the journey as they go on.

Any good lifestyle is a journey. As such, you can expect that your minimalism path will have ups and downs, ins and outs, twists and turns and all sorts of unexpected events. Nothing will go as planned, and in most instances that is the beauty of life itself. These are just some of the things that you can look forward to enjoying during your own minimalist journey.

Knowing that minimalism is a journey is very important. It means that you are not going to go into it thinking that you will master it or that it will all become easier overnight. While it is comprised of many skills, it is not something that you can simply learn and then walk away from. The balance that is required to maintain a minimalist lifestyle takes constant maintenance to ensure that you are not depriving yourself of your basic needs, nor that you are overindulging in things that you do not need. You will always have to maintain this balance using tact, mindfulness, and practice. But, as with any good journey, it is completely worthwhile if you stay committed to the process.

Minimalism is a wonderful opportunity to learn about yourself and the things you love. You gain the ability to become the person you desire to be, and you can have any experience you want in life. The first part to mastering your own mindfulness journey and your experiences is to realize that you will never fully master them. Then, you need to get focused and find ways to stay focused on the purpose behind your journey. Once you have, you will be ready to have any experience you desire in life. The money, time, and resources will be available to you, because you have gotten your priorities straight.

Chapter 2: Perks Of Minimalism And Decluttering, According To Science

Science reveals that accumulating more stuff in your life does not guarantee you happiness. A study done in 2017 determined that clutter is closely linked to procrastination, with people opting not to clear out their homes because they find it cleaning and organizing too much of a burden. The problem is that avoiding household work actually has a negative impact on your mind's well-being. The same study reported that having problems with clutter resulted to an increase in feelings of dissatisfaction among older adults.

Living with clutter, according to another study, also raises your cortisol (stress hormone) levels. It was found that women in cluttered homes had increased cortisol levels all through the day. The same women also disclosed that, as the day progressed, they felt more depressed, and that on top of finding it hard to make the transition from work life to home life, they felt more tired when evening came. Men showed less signs of being bothered by clutter, which explains their lower cortisol levels. With such results, the study suggests the higher sense of responsibility that women have for their home environments, in contrast to men.

Your concentration can also be negatively affected by living in a cluttered home. A Princeton Neuroscience Institute study revealed that being exposed to high levels of visual stimuli prevents the brain from properly focusing and processing information. This is the reason people's mental power and productivity level dip when looking at too many things at the same time.

Benefits of Minimalism and Decluttering

Eliminating clutter from your life can be overwhelming, but you will be reaping plenty of benefits out of it:

Better sleep: If you have ever experienced lying in bed and getting stressed out from staring at either your cluttered closet or towering laundry pile in the hamper, then you must also have experienced hardly getting any rest. A recent study on sleep found a link between lacking sleep and a messy room, especially if the person involved is highly likely to develop a hoarding disorder. The sleeping problem may involve finding it difficult to fall asleep at nighttime and having trouble going back to sleep when awakened.

More focus on goals: Allowing clutter to accumulate means you will be constantly reminded of all the stuff you had to do but failed to follow through. While such a situation may be good in the beginning, such as a yoga mat standing in a corner helps you remember to finally start your stretching routine, it can later on lead to the yoga mat going unused for months until it becomes a form of clutter. Your reason for keeping stuff and living with all that mess could be that you are sure you will finally lose that extra twenty pounds and actually fit into your favorite jeans, or you just know that you will find the time to read all of those old newspapers stacked on the living room floor. But the truth is that those things that you do not really need but are still holding onto will only serve as symbols of guilt and shame instead of being your objects for motivation and inspiration.

Intensified concentration: Having a mess on your home office desk can make getting anything done an absolutely painful chore. But it may surprise you to know that taking the time to get rid of those unnecessary papers and then returning everything you do need in an organized manner can help you get started on your work almost right away. It does not even matter if you are going to be working with an office desk or your bedroom close. Being surrounded by too many things can negatively affect your focusing and information processing ability. A Princeton University study showed that people's task performances differ depending on whether they are working in an organized or a cluttered space. The same study also revealed that when your surroundings have physical clutter, the latter ends up competing for your attention and causes your stress levels to increase and your performance level to go down. Basically, useless stuff only leads your brain to do multitasking, and therefore eliminating it helps transform your mind into a powerful concentrating apparatus.

Increased creativity: While you may believe that a messy studio, desk, or home office helps you work on your tasks work better, it is sensible to think that your creative juices will get going when you are in a clutter-free environment. Having your attention divided between lots of stimuli usually leads to higher stress levels and reduced productivity and creativity.

Eliminating emotional baggage: Having too much stuff is an emotional dilemma you can choose to ignore but will find very difficult to succeed in. You could end up spending days going through them and getting your emotions stirred by all those memories, both the good and the bad. The reality is that how clutter affects you typically does not have anything to do with how much clutter there is. For instance, a former best friend's painting that you hung over your bed can cause you to experience a more intense emotional turmoil than a closet filled with messed up extra towels and sheets. To put it simply, naming something as a form of clutter depends less on how it looks and more on how it makes you feel. If you find yourself feeling less satisfied or inspired in your home, take that as a cue to identifying the things that need to be disposed of. Save yourself from going through the emotional roller coaster and get rid of those items that only weigh you down emotionally.

Effortless money saving: If you think trying to save money is as enjoyable as getting punched in the stomach, you will be surprised to know that practicing the minimalist lifestyle allows you to save money like it is the most natural thing to do in the world. Without even trying, the money you would have spent on impulse buying ends up accumulating in the bank. Because minimalism and decluttering help you get your priorities straight, it becomes easier for you to pass up on buying the latest purse in favor of saving up for that grand vacation with your family. By resisting the relentless call of consumerism, you find yourself gaining additional funds you can use to pursue your dream of getting a new degree, taking up cooking classes, or traveling around the world. Minimalism and decluttering make you realize how sensible and more pleasurable it is to pass up on the feeling of gratification that purchasing the newest gadget brings so that you could funnel your funds on your hobbies instead.

Less stress: The more belongings you have, the more you feel stressed over having to look after them as well as getting them repaired when they get broken or lost. You may be all too familiar with that keys + phone + wallet routine that never fails to take place before you leave for work each morning, or that nonstop checking of your passport and boarding passes as you head through airport security. You may not have control over the necessities, but you do have the power to get rid of your extra possessions in order to eliminate the stress and anxiety that their background buzz brings.

Improved health: Spending less time at the hardware store attempting to outdo your next-door neighbor allows you to find the time to finally pursue your fitness goals. You probably used to constantly be telling yourself that you simply do not have the time to go to the gym, but living the minimalist way now enables you to practice yoga, take up running, or play with your kids at the park.

Chapter 3: The Hoarding Crisis - Why Modern Society Is Focused On Accumulating Material Possessions

We have to explore the idea of hoarding and materialism a lot more in order to truly understand why minimalism is a far greater option. Only when something clicks in your mind, when you really 'get it' can you choose a better option.

Minimalism is an intention, remember. It is something you need to live your life by. You can't half understand it, because your mind will always be in conflict. You have to completely understand it and you have to know that your spirit is in agreement. Only then can you live the life with contentment. Otherwise, you're going to think that you're right, but a voice in your head is going to be saying 'go on, buy it'. You'll always be in conflict and having a war with yourself. There's no fun in that.

By having the full understanding, you'll be able to choose the minimalistic way of life for the right reasons.

So, what is hoarding?

There are two sides to hoarding. One is keeping things and refusing to throw them away because you might need them 'one day', and the other is buying things for the sake of it. Hoarding and shopping addictions are quite closely linked.

You might have a cupboard full of things that you never use, but you refuse to throw them away or donate them to a charity because what if you suddenly need them one day? What if you suddenly wake up on a Thursday morning and need the four vases you have sitting in a cupboard? It's highly unlikely you will ever need those vases but your brain tricks you into thinking that your life will somehow be less meaningful if they are no longer sat in the cupboard.

That is the mindset of a hoarder.

There is nobody in the world who doesn't hoard to some degree when they are not firmly in the minimalistic lifestyle. Everyone who doesn't live the minimalist way hoards a certain amount, and it is usually through bulk buying or buying things that you really don't need.

Why People Become Addicted to Shopping And Accumulating Possessions

Do you consider yourself a shopaholic? Think about it carefully. Becoming addicted to shopping and owning things is a serious condition. Just like becoming addicted to drugs, smoking, alcohol, becoming addicted to purchasing things and accumulating possessions is about dependency.

A person who is addicted to shopping gets a high from the process. They find joy in purchasing something new and taking it home. When they swipe their card and the product goes into a carrier bag to be carried home, they feel on top of the world, and it's a chemical high which can be super-addictive. Of course, as with most highs, it diminishes very quickly, and you're left needing another hit in order to feel that good again.

Between the highs come the lows. You start to realise that you've spent too much money, and you might start hiding credit card bills, or placing your purchases under the bed so that your partner doesn't see them and starts questioning you on why you needed another pair of shoes, another phone, another whatever. Both men and women are equally affected by an addiction to accumulating possessions and shopping. This is not a gender thing, although we tend to focus more on women wanting to buy clothes and shoes; men are equally as prone to purchasing unwanted things in a controllable manner, an addictive manner.

So, why do people become addicted to shopping and accumulating items?

For the same reason that perhaps someone becomes addicted to alcohol or binge eating - the high is so delicious. Once it becomes a continuous cycle, addiction is damaging in so many levels.

Maybe you don't consider yourself to have an addiction, but if you are always drawn to purchasing things and you can't stop yourself, you need to question why you're doing it.

Are you doing it because you're trying to keep up with someone? Are you comparing yourself to someone and purchasing the same items as them in an attempt to 'copy' them or somehow compete? Modern society has become so addicted to 'one-upping' one another that purchasing unneeded items has become almost second nature for so many.

Emotional Causes For Embracing Materialism

Of course, there is a myriad of reasons why someone might get so attracted to materialism, but most of them are emotional. A few potential reasons include:

• A lack of self-confidence and discipline

• Trying to recover from one addiction, and reframing it into another

•Feeling lack in some way, e.g. comparisons to other people and coming up short in your own mind

• Distraction techniques - many people develop an addiction when they are trying not to deal with another issue in their lives, e.g. depression, guilt, or unresolved anger

• Shopping once more as a way of trying to reduce the guilt of the last shopping spree

Materialism does not lead to happiness and it does nothing for confidence. Choosing material things over more deeper connections leads to disconnections in so many areas of life. By addressing the emotional problem at hand, and not trying to avoid it, a person can get away from the grips of consumerism and materialism, but minimalism is a sure fire answer to this problem.

There are a few different types of shopaholics we should mention:

• Emotional shoppers - Those who want to purchase new things because they are feeling distressed emotionally

• Shoppers who are looking for the perfect item - This is a never-ending cycle

• Shoppers who want people to think they're somehow superior - This is a confidence issue, as wanting someone to have a specific view of you is a sign of very low self-worth

• Compulsive shoppers who want to find bargains - This type of shopper is always looking for cut-price items, but in reality, these are not bargains, because you don't need them!

- Cyclic shoppers - These shoppers buy things and take them back, simply to get the hit of purchasing something

Regardless of the type of shopaholic, there is a deep-seated need which is not being addressed, and in order to solve it, a certain amount of soul searching, personal development or even professional help may be necessary.

What We Have Learnt in This Chapter

This chapter has explored the modern day problem of materialism and shopping addictions in greater detail. It is far easier to develop a shopping problem these days than it has ever been before. There is so much focus on owning things and being the one with the flashiest item, the newest piece of technology, that overspending and developing a habit can become all too easy.

In order to escape the grips of materialism, it's vital to understand the reason for needing to own these things in the first place. What are you lacking? Do you feel that you're not good enough? What exactly is driving your need to purchase something?

Once you've understood the reason for your attraction towards hoarding, you can get a birds-eye view of your life circumstances. And that will lead to much better decisions in the journey towards creating a life of fulfillment. Minimalism is the ideal antidote to today's problem of materialism.

Chapter 4: Declutter

Declutter Your Life

Decluttering your physical space can have an amazingly uplifting effect on your mood and feelings. Feng Shui experts claim that buildings and furniture store the memories of events in the form of energy, and that by de-cluttering you can clear the energy of historic traumatic events. Whether or not you put any store in that kind of theory, nobody who has ever de-cluttered a place could deny the positive benefits of increasing the physical space in their environment.

However, physical de-cluttering can also have a cathartic effect on people emotionally. When we let go of things we've been hoarding for a long time, we often let go of emotional memories we've been hanging onto along with them (albeit unconsciously), and so by clearing physical clutter you can clear space in your mind as well as your home.

Clutter though is not only physical. We can also have mental and emotional clutter blocking the flow of energy in our lives, and clearing this out is guaranteed to help improve our emotional health. Examples include undone/unfinished tasks; people/activities that drain you of energy; remaining angry with people; busyness - filling up your schedule with activities you feel duty-bound to do, and leaving no time to nourish your soul and refresh your body.

Some tips for clearing your physical clutter:

• Look at your home and identify the areas that need decluttering. Break it down into small tasks that can be managed over a period of time, rather than one big project to be done in a day. Start small with everyday places like the kitchen table and build momentum towards the areas you avoid because the idea of tackling them is just overwhelming.

• Go through your stuff and for each item ask yourself Do I love it? Do I need it? Do I use it? If you can answer yes to any of them, it stays. If it is no to all, then it goes.

• Divide everything into four piles: Keep, Recycle, Donate and Dump. As soon as you are done, remove the items that are not staying straight away and deliver them to their new destination.

• Once your big clear out is done, avoid a new build up by clearing out little and often.

Tips for clearing your Mental/Emotional Clutter:

• Make a list of anything you have been procrastinating over, and ask yourself why you have been putting it off. What can you tackle and what can you let go of? When you are clear on what you definitely has to be done, make a roadmap and get to it.

• Stop worrying too much. There is nothing constructive about worrying – it will not help you avoid the outcome you are worrying about and it'll destroy your ability to enjoy the present. When a worrying thought arises, quash it straight away and sing along with me "Everything's going to be alright…" Focus your energy on what you would like to happen instead.

• Follow through on promises and commitments. When you have said you will do something but you keep putting it on the long finger, it drains you of energy. If you cannot or do not want to see them through, then be upfront about it and withdraw your promise.

• Let go of anger. When somebody hurts you badly, it is a normal response to feel anger, and to not want to forgive. However, anger is bad for your health, both physical and emotional, so it is actually in your interests to let it go and forgive the other person. Forgiving them does not mean you have to welcome them back into your life with open arms, it just means letting go of the memory of what they have done to you and the feelings that go with it. Maybe the other person does not deserve forgiveness, but do not you deserve to move on and leave the pain behind?

• Say no to people and activities that drag you down. Instead, surround yourself with people who uplift you and do things that make you feel great!

As with your physical clear out, do not make this a once-off project. Develop clutter free habits in every area of your life, and you will enjoy an easier flow through life on a continuous basis.

Five Benefits of Daily Decluttering

You can reconnect with people, activities, and important information that you may have been neglecting.

You get to spend a few minutes each day evaluating what you have in your life and whether you want to keep it in your life.

You will feel less stressed and if you de-clutter on a daily basis than if you wait for the piles (and relationship issues) to build up.

You will have more room in your life for new opportunities if you keep your life and environment clutter free.

You will experience the joy of knowing you have your life under control.

Where to Start:

Declutter your relationships. Call someone you have been meaning to call. Send a note card or holiday greeting with an invitation to get together after the holidays.

Declutter your personal environment. Clear out your closet, work desk, kitchen, holiday decorations. Take a look around and see what stuff is getting in your way-- then doing something about it!

Declutter your relationship with God. Talk to Him, spend time with Him, dust off your Bible and Bible study books. Move them to a convenient location so you can spend a few minutes with the God.

Declutter your financial situation. Balance your checkbook, create a budget, choose and start working a plan to become debt free or increase your savings and investment portfolio.

Declutter your health. Clean the junk food out your cabinets and refrigerator, locate your walking shoes, and call your doctor to schedule your next physical.

Tips for Success:

Start small. Do not let your feelings of overwhelm let you down. Pick a corner of your desk, one shelf in a closet, or one person to contact.

Put on music or listen to an audio book while you work.

Set a timer and stop when the bell sounds.

Use 5 or 10-minute blocks of time while waiting for the coffee to brew, the laundry to finish.

Share your success with a friend.

Take before and after pictures.

Experience the pleasure of small bursts of clutter-free living. Build the momentum.

Reward yourself when a major task is completed.

Declutter Before Packing to Move

Decluttering before packing is an important aspect when preparing to move - because it allows you to decide what you will need for the new house, what you will have room for, and what you need.

The most important thing to remember when decluttering is that you will be making room and getting rid of emotional baggage, whilst lowering your moving bills. An average four-person house requires at least an eight-ton van to move, whilst a house that does not declutter might need twice that!

De-cluttering can be considered essential or heartless - but either way, moving house is one of the best times to do a proper de-clutter - in fact sometimes, it is the only 'spring clean' that some people do. In addition, while it is always good to hang onto things of sentimental value, do you really need a newspaper from 1985 with an article about something that you needed to follow up within a week of the printing?

Get rid of any papers that you don't need (though keep all important documentation) - consider donating any magazines, books, old toys or clothes in good condition to a local charity - or sell them on Ebay or similar, to make some cash.

These donations and sales make mental and space sense - you are not wasting perfectly good items you will probably never use again, and you could sell the really good condition items in a variety of places. You could hold a yard sale, or garage or even a car boot sale - or if you have enough time, auction them online, either via a recognized site, or through your own website, if you have the know how - getting rid of the things you don't need is both very freeing and releasing, and can actually generate you some extra money for the move. You could even sell off surplus office, or craft supplies, if you have them spare, making your home office move leaner, and easier.

Declutter Checklist

One of the fastest ways to increase the success of your life / business / work is to do a thorough house cleaning. Sounds silly? It works. By clearing out the physical clutter and debris in your working area, you will correspondingly clear out mental clutter that prevents you from manifesting abundance. In addition to this, by disposing of unneeded items that no longer serve you, we are making space that can be used for new items to replace them. The important point is that you concentrate on developing new and more effective ways of doing, finding new markets, and streamline your working area so as to get the maximum results from your freelancing.

Here are some guidelines for clearing the clutter from your life:

1. Check your computer. Delete duplicate files and files that you have not used in a year. If you have a mass of documents in the My Documents folder, this is time to organize them and classify them under folders. Devise a tracking system for your queries. Review your ideas and see which ones can be developed into good articles. Delete the rest.

2. How much of the contents of your desk have not been used in over a year? Out they go. Be ruthless. Remember, you are holding in mind that your success is on its way and you need to make room for it.

3. Check your bookcases. You can extend the one-year rule a bit here, but you must be realistic with yourself. Are you actually going to make use of these things in your work? Throw away what you must, sell

what you can and give the rest to a charity.

4.Start bringing a higher level of order into your life. Are there people to whom you owe a letter? Have you balanced your checkbook? This is the time to either create or refine your "to do" list and make it stick. Carry it around with you and add to it as you think of new items. You will find that many of the items that you add to your list will directly affect your level of success. The reason for this is that success flows in the presence of order. Just as water is disturbed into rapids in the presence of major outcroppings of rocks, so is the flow of success disrupted by the disorder of cluttered schedules, incomplete duties and commitments. You may note that it is very rare that a prosperous individual allows their affairs to be chaotic.

Not all of this has to happen in one weekend. In order to make it work effectively, daily progress should be happening. Choose one cabinet to clean out per day or one letter to write. Make your progress towards greater order a tangible thing that you can recognize. The results will be well worth it.

Chapter 5: The Promises Of Consumerism

Consumerism has always been confused with happiness. There is always a tendency towards materialism and greed, which turns out to be the most significant human weakness. It is now a century old modern phenomenon. In the 1920's America, advertisers purposefully linked ownership to happiness in the minds of the public. They got help from experts in the field of psychology. A Freudian psychoanalyst, Ernst Ditcher assisted by advertisers said that to a certain extent, the wants and needs of people need to be continually stirred up.

This strategy is still prevalent. Today, an exotic vacation, an iPad, or the latest handbag have become equivalent to respect. Some brands of beer are a symbol of a sense of community and friendship. A large house means status and proof of how rich you are. These are ideas instilled in the minds of clients by advertisers who profit when we buy what we don't need.

They are so successful at using our selfish desires for ownership that today they market buying and being happy as the same thing. Self-gratification is seen as the purpose of life, and buying things is the only way there. We don't spend time thinking about this, but most of us subconsciously buy into it.

The one reason why this issue persists is that our culture is consumption oriented. Consumerism is like the air we breathe, and it is invisible. We are not aware of how influenced we are by the philosophy that we must keep buying if we want to be happy. It feels normal to us because our inner desires equal the external messages. We go along with this philosophy, maybe occasionally feeling awkward or doubtful about the meaning of it all.

We have to intentionally find our blind spot and examine what we have ignored to overcome our consumerist inclinations. The magnitude of consumerist propaganda should be measured and observed to know how deeply it has penetrated public discourse and our own perspectives. Primarily, we have to admit that we are influenced by it. For only then can we stand against it and stop it from affecting our life. It is not an easy thing to do, but the benefits are so worth it. We get to discover more reliable sources of happiness.

For instance, consider how pervasive this perspective is. We have streets lined with malls and stores. We gauge our wellbeing as a nation based on trade deficits, gross domestic profits, rate of inflation, and consumer confidence. Every single corner of the Nation has been commercialized, including national parks. We choose our political leaders single-handedly based on the promises they make on what they can do for the health of the economy. The dollar signs and square footage are the symbols of the American dream. To make this resistance much more complicated, the best minds of this generation use every mechanism to create commodities that can turn us into even greedier customers.

It just takes one single click of a button to purchase something. Due to the elevated opportunity for personal data collection with technology, target marketing has helped businesses become harder to avoid. Gone are the days where they just knew our name, gender, age, and marital status. Today they know our net worth, our shopping habits, our favorite books, movies, and personal preferences. Where we spend, how and on what is all known to these corporations. Our smartphones and Internet browser history collect every single data recorded. It is used to exploit our weaknesses every day.

In a way, marketers have more information about us than we have of ourselves. They feed into our insecurities and inadequacies. Our passions are hijacked by society and directed towards materialism. However, at the end of life, nobody wished that they had more things. That is because consumption never completely delivers on its promises of fulfillment and happiness. In its place, they steal our results and freedom to tap into our insatiable desire for more. It brings regret and burden and distracts us from the real things that give us joy.

Please do not jump to the conclusion that resisting consumerism in itself will bring you happiness. An absence of something is just nothingness. What matters is how we replace it, and we have to take small steps towards it. Resisting consumerism can help us from fundamental deception and even see a possibility of real satisfaction, whatever meaning that holds to each of us.

This book will highlight specific areas of consumerism, spotting its impacts where you might not have noticed before and exposed its true form:

- The materialistic attitude towards ownership that you may have because of the generation you belong to

- How success is defined according to the world, you are in

- How you are manipulated by marketers when you shop

Song Dong, a Chinese artist, displayed his collection of household items, titled Waste, which had been owned by his late mother. The installation involved an inventory of personal belongings: pots, cups, toothpaste, shirts, basins, skipping rope, stuffed animals, pieces of string, rice bowls, neckties, ten thousand items in total. All the items were crammed into her home in Beijing, which was only a few hundred square feet.

The first emotional response was perplexity. Why would someone keep twelve empty tubes of toothpaste or several pieces of string? The second response was wonder. How did it fit into a small house? Third response: revulsion. What a terrible way to live! However, in the end, we end up with gratitude. It was clear that the exhibit was demonstrating the ideology of an entire era of people living in China during wartime, starvation, rationing, constant shortage of goods, and expulsion. For the artists' mother, possessing any worldly goods meant survival. What seemed to be a hoarding match was, in reality, an effective response to external devastation.

If you are from a developed nation, you never had to deal with economic or global insecurity. Therefore, you don't have the need to hold on to everything that you come across in preparation for raiding or famine. You have the freedom to choose less, and that is a privilege too, and we should be grateful for it. Song Dongs exhibit is a sharp contrast to how people respond to different living conditions and material possessions these days.

In the broadest sense generation analysis is not exactly science. However, it gives you deep insights that help with self-understanding. Identify your generation and start to understand the different influences and outlooks towards consumption and accumulation.

- 1928-1945 are the Silent Generation
- 1946-1964 are the Baby Boomer Generation
- 1965-1980 are the Generation X
- 1981-2000 are the Millennial Generation

Consumerism and the Silent Generation

This generation was part of World War II and The Great Depression.

Their generational views were waste not, want not. They were people who had items that were built to last for ages. They grew up in an America with drought and high unemployment followed by the harshest wars the world has ever seen and to top that, rationing. They had to live frugally and if possible, save what they had.

Today the silent generation survivors are in their seventies and eighties. They are starting to move to smaller living spaces by choice or by necessity; however, always with a heavy heart. This is why organizations such as National Association for Senior Move Managers are essential. Downsizing is difficult, physically, and mentally since they lived in the same places for several years.

Minimizing is not an advantage but also a necessity. It is essential to understand how you need to avoid the appeal of consumerism. The lesson to have a simpler life from youth and resisting the mainstream ideals towards ownership will give you an unburdened life, which is peaceful and rewarding.

Consumerism and the Baby Boomer Generation

This is the generation that was born right after World War II; America encountered severe housing shortages for the men and women returning from service and a very high birth rate. This created a sudden expansion in the home building section in suburban areas. Baby boomers were raised in large number in the suburbs that came with the cultural forces.

They benefitted from the era of prosperity. Women were working outside their homes, and families become dual income for the first time in history. Post-war optimism instilled opportunity and stability. They became consumers of the first order. This generation is now established, grown, and on its own. They are soon to retire.

They might not be comfortable with the idea of consumerism, but they have started to see its benefits. If you belong to this generation, at this point in your life, you are questioning if buying is equal to happiness. Even though you lived half of your life in a large house in the suburbs, accompanied by comforts of a past life. Perhaps you are thinking about the importance of experiences over possessions. Maybe you are emphasizing your legacy rather than adding to a pile of commodities. If so, you are on the right track.

Consumerism and Generation X

Generation X is referred to as individualistic, cynical, and self-involved survivalist. In several ways, they are caught between consumerism at its most uncontrolled realities of what owning too much really means. Generation X grew up in working families with disposable income but with little time and energy for their children. They came of age during the technological revolution. This made the world more mobile. Owing to individualistic pursuits and distrust of governing bodies, Gen-X will have an average of seven career changes during their lifetime.

Kids have a way of changing personalities. Moreover, Gen Xers are now middle-aged and dealing with children of all ages. They have become helicopter parents. The baby boomer grandparents who are used to expressing affection through gifts, Gen-X homes are overrun with the mess. If you are a part of this generation, you days of maximum pay benefits are numbered. You also know how over accumulation has brought the worst things to you. Control it before it's too late.

Consumerism and the Millennial Generation

Minimalism is the natural way to live for this generation. They are the first generation after the technological boom. Their world is smaller and connected at the same time. Coffee shops can turn out to be offices; the new competition is collaboration and stability.

This generation is very environmentally conscious of all age groups, and this affects their buying habits. There are opportunities like the sharing economy, where assets are not owned by individuals but shared communally. Ownership has been replaced by access.

The Internet serves as a worldwide flea market. Any product purchased will be available to you in the flick of a button.

Another important fact is that this generation has graduated from college and entered workplaces in the middle of the great recession. Student loans and underemployment has left some millennials with little to no income. Millennials are in a position in life where they can choose to live minimally better than everybody else.

It is important to note how casual our relationship with consumer culture is. It should also be recognized that all generations in America are susceptible to confusing excess with success.

Chapter 6: Lessening The Clutter

Less is always more because it makes you very aware of everything that you have. You can see it and it isn't covered up by layers of stuff that is superfluous. If you have a spare room, ask yourself if the furniture in it is all necessary or whether it's too big for the room. Often we inherit items and simply place them in the spare room because we don't have any other place for it. Then, when we have guests, we panic about making the room look good. It is a far better idea to keep the room neat and tidy all of the time as you can use this space for other things. For example, if you want to practice yoga or you want a quiet space to be to do computer work, there's nothing to stop you enjoying the spare room if it isn't cluttered with stuff. It also makes cleaning so much easier.

The idea is to take a notebook into each room of your house and be totally honest about what adds value to your life and what does not. People find it hard to let go of things, but at the end of the day, I have seen so many people thrilled with the results of decluttering that I know it's a worthwhile task and when you stop letting your ownership of things dictate the quality of your life, the quality automatically goes up. You create more space in your home. It's easier to clean. You don't have things that remind you of spending money or wasting money on things you can never use. How many of the clothes in your closet are actually ones that you wear? There's a huge guilt trip attached to keeping clothes in the hope that one day you will slim down and fit into them. Believe me, if you ever do get to that stage, you won't want those old clothes, because you will have created a new image and going out to buy new clothes is much more likely. Why face that failure every day of your life as you struggle through the piles of clothes that no longer fit you?

The thing that we all do is get fooled by advertisements. We see that magic gadget that will do the hard work we don't want to do and we buy into the dream, only to find that it's actually not worth the effort because you have all different kinds of obligations attached to using these gadgets. For example, cleaning up the mixer after you have made cakes is harder than cleaning up a traditional bowl. The deep fat fryer we hoped would hide all the grease just harbors it and every time we open it, we are reminded that we haven't bothered cleaning it. An air fryer does the frying without the tears and takes up much less space. What you are doing is not depriving yourself of things you need, but you are rethinking what you need so that only things that add joy to your life find room within the walls of your home.

Closets that are full of things mean that you don't even have room to hide your clutter anymore. These are spaces that you need to sort out. If you find, for example, that you have a pile of paperwork sorted into boxes, why keep that system going. Not only do you have to deal with each piece of paper that comes into the home, but you also obligate yourself to store them. The option is to go paperless. That doesn't mean that you don't have access to your paperwork, because you can access past bills online, but it does mean that you make the utilities store all of the paper! The same can be done with your bank account.

Photographs and mementos may be important to you but set them all out on a table and work out which act as artwork and which can be digitized so that you have them on memory sticks and can access them when you need to, instead of having to dust around them all of the time.

As your family grows, so do your possessions. Take a look at what is superfluous. You may have needed that tiny chair for your son and perhaps you have been keeping it for your grandson, but why does it need to clutter your home? Put it away in the loft or the cellar and wrap it up so that it doesn't get harmed in the process of storage. You need to have in your home things that are current to your lifestyle now, rather than all of this stuff that relates to other times.

I wouldn't mind betting that as technology has advanced, you have bought into the dream and perhaps have a drawer full of old technology. This serves you no purpose at all except to remind you that you were perhaps a little frivolous in your spending. If you don't want something, get rid of it. That rainy day isn't going to happen and all this stuff is merely filling your home to brimming with your past failures. You have to understand that too much exposure to social media pressure and advertisements on the TV usually means that you are not better off buying into the dream. You are better off deciding upon the best phone for you and sticking to that decision, instead of always wanting to upgrade.

The things that you have in your home that are of no use to you should go.

Minimalism isn't about depriving yourself. It's about making choices that fit with your life. It isn't about saving money frugally. It's about using the money that you have to maximize your lifestyle. Things that you buy that have a week's novelty are really not going to add value to your life. All the hype in the world doesn't mean they are going to change who you are and that's where people go wrong. The latest iPhone – does it do more than the older model? It probably does, but are the new features important to your life? If they are not, then there's little point in spending money on something you will never really need.

You have the mindset now and in this chapter, we encouraged you to face the truth about what you own. In the next chapter, it's time to live up to the dream and feel the liberation of getting rid of junk.

Chapter 7: The Initial Steps To A Minimalistic Way Of Life

If you resemble many people, then you're most likely living a way of life that is a long way from minimalism. The odds are that each and every single surface area is covered in unnecessary clutter and that you have a lengthy list of things you desire which you plan to spend your cash on and feel like you can't rather pay for the lifestyle that you desire or feel you should have.

You have actually discovered why this is an issue and how it can make you dissatisfied. Now it's time to begin finding a solution for it!

Follow these actions to start your journey towards a genuinely minimalistic way of life.

Decrease Your Clutter

We have actually utilized the word 'clutter' a lot already, and that's due to the fact that it actually is among the most significant issues. Minimalism does not indicate not having wonderful things; it indicates not having the things you do not truly require or desire.

As an experiment, I want you to go into any room in your home and head over to one of the surfaces-- whether that's a bedroom cabinet, a desk or a windowsill. Now, have a look at those objects on display and get rid of 60% of them.

This is going to feel off initially. It is going to feel as though you're removing things you actually like or that you're leaving that surface too sporadic. However, go with it.

What you'll discover is that far from looking worse, getting rid of those things really makes your surface area look a LOT better and that minimalism gives area for your belongings to breathe, and it makes them stand out more. What's more, is that it exposes the real surface beneath and gets rid of the visual 'noise' out of the corner of your eye, which can really wind up producing a great deal of tension.

What's remaining is now the premium 40% of your things. That suggests that what you have actually left behind are going to be things that you truly like. It implies that the typical quality of what's on that surface area is going to increase considerably. And those couple of things that stay are going to state far more about you and are going to bring in a lot more attention-- rather than simply blending into a congested mess.

The very best part, however, is that when you then come to clean up that surface area, you are going to have the ability to do so by merely getting rid of 3 or 4 things, and after that, wiping. This has now ended up being a 3-minute task, rather than a 10-minute task. And picture what is going to occur when you apply that identical reasoning to all the other surface areas in your home!

Now go and do the identical thing for all those other surface areas in your room!

Get rid of Boxes

The reason that getting rid of clutter is so effective is that it offers you psychological space. Our brains are developed to take notice of contrast and things that stick out, and they do this by discharging tiny quantities of stress hormone. The more noise and clutter there is in an area, the more there is for our brains to handle. This could be frustrating, and after a long, tough day at work, it makes it extremely hard to unwind and loosen up.

The reality that they add more work just further imposes the truth that an abundance of things does not contribute to your area.

The identical goes for a variety of other things that you most likely do not recognize are resulting in you being stressed. Case in point: boxes that you have beneath your bed or atop your closet. This most likely appears like a fantastic location for storage that is out of the way and assists you to keep more things. However, the truth is that it is going to create visual clutter and work again.

For starters, boxes underneath the bed and on the closet get terribly dusty unless they have a lid. However, more significantly, they once again are going to occupy your mind by using up space and by getting rid of those important areas of 'space' that make a room feel much larger and much less heavy.

Simply attempt taking the boxes out from under the bed and atop the closet and see if this produces a more peaceful and tidy-looking environment. Do the identical for things atop bookshelves, beneath coffee tables, and crammed behind couches.

And once again, simply think how simpler the cleaning is going to be.

It's time to begin thinking of the negative area in your house as being just as crucial-- if not more crucial-- than the clutter that encompasses it.

Dealing with Cables

Another essential suggestion is to consider your cable management. Today, you most likely have cables running beneath desks, throughout the floor, and almost anywhere else.

Can you guess what these do? That's right: they develop more visual clutter! And they make your house appear a lot messier and chaotic than it most likely is. There are terrific cable management options, which vary from utilizing boxes to save your cables, to connecting them to the underside of desks and the rears of screens. Get imaginative, and you can make a lot more space!

One In, One Out

Among the very best things you may do to keep an uncluttered house is to present guidelines that are going to assist you to keep a more minimalistic design.

One such guideline is 'one in, one out.' This just suggests that each time you purchase a brand-new product, you have to select one you have to do away with. This is going to assist you to keep a reasonable variety of things in your house that never ever become overwhelming, and it is going to assist you to spare cash-- particularly seeing as you can sell the things that you do not require in order to get cash off of the brand-new item. It makes an area for your brand-new thing right away, and it additionally pushes you to think much harder about the important things that you really desire.

This seems like a severe guideline, but once you begin to see and feel the advantages of living a more minimalist way of life, you'll more than happy to do it!

Removing Things

If you follow all of these pointers, then you're going to discover that you're dealing with a great deal of things. This could be an unpleasant procedure; however, there is an art to getting it right.

Initially, you are going to do a huge 'de-clutter' and remove a great deal of things rapidly. This is going to aid you to reset your life so that you have an excellent beginning point to work from.

The primary step is to throw away boxes of things that you have actually been keeping in storage that you never ever utilize. The guideline that is typically provided here is to throw away any box that you have not gone into in the last 3 months (you 'd marvel how many that includes!). Also, get rid of clothing that you have not used in 3 months.

Another idea is to remove these things quickly. If you have items you believe you can get a great deal of cash for, then these are worth selling. However, all else you ought to offer to charity stores or throw away.

It's an error to leave things in bags, to let family and friends go through them, or to attempt and sell every last thing. This not just produces a lot more tension as you need to go through all the things you own (hence implying a great deal of individuals are going to put it off and refrain from doing it!), however, it additionally develops the temptation to reconsider and take things back. This is not the objective of the game!

Chapter 8: The Transition

At this juncture, you think you can become a minimalist. The benefits sound wonderful, and you want to live a happier, freer life. But, how can you transition from the habits and lifestyle you have to the minimalist one?

There are numerous answers to the above question. Not one of the answers is the "right" one. Each person has to transition in a way that makes the most sense to them. You might look at the twenty-one-- day steps that are outlined below and know you can keep to the schedule, but what happens after? Are you the type of person that can continue on that minimalism path even if you encounter problems?

A key element to transitioning into the minimalist mindset is knowing your strengths and weaknesses. Courtney Carver believes there are three types of categories new minimalists fit into. But, you cannot quantify it to just three because everyone has a personality, separate from the rest of the world. We are individuals because of these traits. Do not think you have to conform to Carver's three categories.

The first category is the person ready to go, ready to become a minimalist and declutter their home. The second is the type of person who feels they have limited space, not that they have too much to fill the space they have. The third is interested but does not know how to begin the process.

The law of averages says a person who rushes into decisions will falter at some point during the process. The individual who takes their time, thinks it through, and slowly begins to become a minimalist often succeeds where others do not. Again, there is no hard and fast rule about how you change your life and adopt the Japanese art of minimalism. Do what works for you, correct the transition process if something does not work, and realize that you may have to work at it for a while.

Minimalism is a lifestyle change, not an overnight transition.

This is the point where you need to assess reality.

- Do you have a spouse?

- Do you have children?

- Are there other family members who are part of your life or that you live with?

- Do you take a radical change with ease or does it cause fear?

- Are you willing to experiment before you find the level of minimalism you are comfortable with?

- Do you know what makes you happy?

- Are you willing to accept that you will continue to try and define your life, so there is no end point to reach with minimalism?

How you answer the above questions is going to define what you are willing to try and do to become a minimalist. For people who have a spouse, the husband or wife will need to accept your need to change and have less to gain more. If children are involved, then you are teaching them a lesson, but a drastic change may not be possible.

Children learn from their parents. Seeing an extravagant lifestyle that is suddenly reduced to a few favorite things, with fewer expensive vacations or presents, will result in a need for time to adjust. But, the good news is you can teach them better values as you make this transition and help them see why you felt a change was necessary.

Seven Possible Steps

The following are seven suggestions you might consider to begin the transition of becoming a minimalist.

Write down a plan based on reality.

Find one place in your home that is clutter-free. This is the room that never becomes a mess. It is the room to start with, and then you can eventually make other rooms just as clutter-free.

Get rid of duplicate items, whether it is clothing or photographs.

Dress using less clothing and alternate how you wear them in combination.

Travel with fewer items. Do you need a bathing suit each day you are in the Caribbean? Are you going to need more than three changes of clothes for a week on a cruise, when you have a way to wash them? You can travel with less.

Adapt the meals you eat, such as using the crockpot more, as making meals that contain all nutritional value with fewer steps is possible. You can simplify meals to gain more time with family.

Save at least $1,000. This is the end step in this process of transition. You can do this by changing your shopping habits for clothing, new home items, and food. When you are buying less, it is possible to save more.

You may be a person that needs more steps or more elaborate considerations. You may also need a plan that is less easy to forget about.

Discover Twenty-One Steps

Psychologists believe that your mind needs twenty-one days to form new habits. To break the cycle you are in, you want to make certain your brain can adapt. This idea can also be applied to becoming a minimalist with a twenty-one step plan done over a period of twenty-one days to help your brain restructure. You may need longer. You might require less time. But, if you want to feel less stress, more confidence, and overall success, then trying for a twenty-one-day change is helpful. Better than anything else, you can use this concept for dieting, meal planning, and minimalism, so it is not just a concept rooted solely in changing your mindset to be a minimalist.

Decide to become a minimalist.

Plan your steps to make this happen.

Start packing what you know you do not need.

Organize the essential items.

Assess the things that give you pause—you might have a sentimental attachment but can still get rid of it.

Examine the fear you feel for your new lifestyle.

Look at the relationships in your life and who is helping you.

Believe that changes can be made.

Grow as a person.

Examine everything so far and see how you feel.

Get rid of the trash.

Start selling items to others who will value them.

Donate what cannot be sold.

Digitize aspects of your life to declutter, such as photographs.

Examine what is left and continue reducing what you can.

Target your car—can you get rid of it or own a more minimalist vehicle?

Can you move to a smaller home?

What can you change at work to declutter and minimalize?

Are there areas of your health you can target?

 Do you have too many electronics? Can you change how you watch TV?

Now you have more time. Organizing and decluttering your life has just provided you with TIME. How will you enjoy it?

These twenty-one steps help you rethink your current life. They allow you to consider the possibilities and make a move toward a happier lifestyle. But, they are not set in stone. You might begin digitizing your photographs before you decide to trash things. Make your transition plan based on who you are, your strengths, and your current commitments.

Your Psychology

What type of personality do you have? Do you think you do better with a few guidelines or every step written out? When you transition into the minimalist mindset, you must know who you are.

Take a look at your life as it is now. What if you were given six months to move out of your home? What if you had to move four times in three years? A lot of times when you look at a situation with a different perspective, it is easier to see how you can become a minimalist, but do you start regaining things in your life once it begins to settle down?

One family has dealt with several struggles in a short period of five years. It started with a move due to health issues, which turned into four moves in three years for one of the family members. Another went through a bankruptcy, divorce, and two years of a battle over children simply for one parent to "win" against the other. Now this family faces another move, with six months to make it happen. For some people, their strength may be gone, but for others, it is the time where each family member rallies to ensure the best possible outcome.

You never know what you will do until you are faced with a situation. If you need something enough, you will find a way to make it happen.

So, begin your transition by assessing what your life has been like, how it has shaped you, and the potential changes you can gain.

What is the hardest event in your life that you have had to face? There is no right or wrong answer. For one person, it might be the loss of a pet, and for another person, it is wondering if this is the year he or she will become paralyzed due to genetic health disorders.

When you faced that difficult event, how did you handle it? Looking back, were there things you could have done better? Going back to the example of the family above, the wife and her two children had to face losing the male of their household. The wife lost a spouse and the children lost a father too early due to onset dementia. One adult child could not be there due to a troubled marriage and two children. The other child never thought she had enough strength to watch her father die slowly, day by day. The wife was not going to leave his side, but she got lost in the loss, unable to focus on anyone else's loss of this same person.

We all react differently to major life events, and, because they are the most trying, they also tell us the most about our personality. You may think you have hit rock bottom until yet another thing tries to strike you down, and you realize life is not all that bad because there are things you still value.

The point is, you will need to assess who you are to know your current limitations and discover your true limits as you work toward a minimalist lifestyle. Right now, you may think, "I do not know how to transition" or "How can I keep to this schedule if something else happens?" The answer is that you will find it when you get to that point.

The move into a minimalist lifestyle is as much about the journey as it is about meeting the goals you set.

If you can remember the above statement, then you can transition to a new lifestyle based on your current psychological traits. You will learn more about yourself as you begin your journey. Look forward to the coming changes.

Embrace what you discover.

You are ready for the next section. You are prepared to start the practical application of the concepts that will move you into a minimalist lifestyle. Be strong, get back up and on track when you falter, and enjoy journeying through minimalism to reach your goals. You are capable of making an impact.

Chapter 9: The Process Of Decluttering

Decluttering the soul is, without a doubt, a difficult thing. To increase your chances of success, it is important that you follow some proven steps. These ensure that you do not skip something crucial along the way. In addition, they break down the decluttering process into easily manageable parts.

Step 1: Define Your Ideal Life

The first step in decluttering your soul is defining what you consider to be the ideal life. You need to know what you consider as most important to you. With this clarity, you will be able to purge everything that might distract you from those important things.

How do you know what matters in life?

You must take a moment and reflect. There are two tricks I like to use. And they take advantage of the power of imagination. The brain cannot differentiate between imagination and reality. Here is the first trick:

- Sit comfortably (anywhere you know you will be comfortable and not get disturbed) and close your eyes.

- Imagine that you have $1 million in your account. With that amount of money, you would afford to live a comfortable life for many years. So you are clearly not in a rush for food, shelter, or other necessities of life. This means you can focus your life on things that truly matter to you.

- Think of the kind of lifestyle you would lead if in a situation like this. Would you focus on traveling the world? Would you spend more time with your family? The trick here is to ensure that you are staying clear of things that promote consumerism.

Another trick is the deathbed test. Here is how you can use it:

- Imagine that you are on your deathbed. Now reflect on the things you have done so far in your life.

- Do they make you feel that you lived life the way you wanted? Was working 15 hours a day really worth it? Was buying trendy gadgets really worth it?

- If you are not proud of some of the things you have been doing, then those things are not essential. If you had a chance to live your life again, what would you do differently?

These two tricks will put your life into focus. Without the demands of everyday life, you will define what really matters to you. And this will help you define your ideal life.

Step 2: Focus on One Thing at a Time

To declutter your soul successfully, you must focus on one thing at a time. If you are looking at your goals, pick each goal and justify its existence. If focusing on feelings, consider each feeling individually. You should zoom in on everything that happens in your life.

That will make the decluttering process less intimidating. And it will ensure for a thorough declutter. Here is a set of questions you need to ask yourself to justify the things you do or have:

- Does this thing get me close to the kind of life I dream to live?

- Does this make me the type of person who I aspire to be?

- What are the effects this thing has had on me?

- How different would my life be if I did not have this thing?

These questions will help you determine what is important and what is not.

Step 3: Purge the Non-Essentials

Now that you know what matters and what doesn't, you can remove all that keeps you from living the kind of life you want. If it is toxic relationships that seem to be the problem, simply stop seeing those people and spend more time developing your fruitful relationships. If it is a long schedule bringing clutter, then trim it.

Purging non-essential things is not easy. You will feel at a loss to not indulge in something you had been accustomed to. You will think your life will be difficult without this thing. Humans are hardwired to fear change. That's because change lives in the future. And that future brings uncertainty.

But you must realize that you cannot grow if you do not seek change. You cannot improve your life or get happier if you are unwilling to move away from your present conditions.

Here are a few tips to guide you:

Start small – you may be tempted to purge lots of things at once to make up for the time you had not been a minimalist. But this is a recipe for disaster. If you employ way too many changes, you will overwhelm yourself. Your brain will not be able to cope with the sudden change of lifestyle. And it will urge you to go back to your old ways.

So, take baby steps. Declutter just one area of your life at a time. For example, start with your schedule and keep it clutter-free for a few weeks. This will allow you to get used to the habit of having a minimalist schedule. When you are done with that, declutter your goals. When you are finished with that, declutter your feelings, and so on.

Of course, this will take you time. But you must know that you are trying to build a lifestyle that will last your lifetime.

Track your progress – most of us are good at starting things. But along the way, we get distracted and give up. This is why it is important to track your progress. Have you managed to declutter your schedule in the way you said you were going to do it? Have you gotten rid of all toxic relationships in your life?

If the goal is to declutter your schedule, then look at it every day to ensure that it is minimalistic. Without this, you will likely lose your way and stop practicing minimalism.

Review your accomplishments – from time to time, sit back to just reflect how far you have come in your minimalistic journey. How do you feel now that you have decluttered your soul? Would you want to go back to your old ways? Obviously, the answer will be "no."

Reviewing keeps you motivated to stick to minimalism. In addition, it convinces you to also declutter other areas of your soul. You become a true minimalist.

Chapter 10: The Benefits Of Minimalism

Minimalism is a positive approach to putting a halt to the greed that surrounds us. We are encumbered by a society that thrives wittingly on the amassment of things.

By embracing the minimalist lifestyle, one can take out the unneeded, the pile of junk, and pay attention to what is genuinely necessary.

People who have accepted the minimalist lifestyle recognize that the paybacks are enormous and completely satisfying.

The benefits of minimalism are quite endless; we'll focus on a few:

Mental Clarity

The connection between our personal belongings and our mental, responsive wellbeing is often undermined. Nevertheless, the bond between them is unquestionable.

Studies show that there is a noticeable boost in clearness of mind and peacefulness when actions such as simply clearing out a closet are undertaken. If you think it over, when was the last time you took the time to go through your storage space or the attic? When was the last time you reorganized all of the stuff you had piled up in those spaces? After you did go through them, what was the predominant feeling you had as soon as you were done?

It was certainly a feeling of ease, as though you had a weight taken off your shoulders, and maybe you expended a small amount of energy in the past just thinking about the junk you had piled up, simply clearing them out gave you a genuine sense of calm. This feeling of calm, tranquility, and relief is more than just feeling; it is well founded and backed by scientific research.

The truth is, when we hold on so tightly to quantifiable properties, we unintentionally but inadvertently generate an enormous amount of stress; this is because of the underlying phobia that we all possess when it comes to the fear of losing them. By making your life simpler, it becomes remarkably more comfortable to drop your affection for things, and in the long run create a tranquil, peaceful mind. The less stuff you worry your mind over, the more tranquility you garner.

Tick the appropriate box for each remark

	REMARK	YES	MAYBE	NO
1	I get happier whenever I clean my storage space			
2	I feel my stress levels go down every time I do some spring cleaning			
3	Whenever my mind is clear, I tend to be more generally effective			

| 4 | I think my mental liberty affects my physical outlook | | |

Value- added Health

Our health is no laughing matter. A lifestyle that breeds stress, heaps, and piles of junk, which eventually leads to uncleanliness, will inadvertently affect one's health. You may think that ridding yourself of a few items might not so much as change your health condition; but looking a little closer, you would notice that acts, such as clearing your schedule of unnecessary commitments can do wonders for your overall being.

Over-commitment is hazardous to our lives, and the quest to please other people beyond our actual ability keeps us well within the ditch.

Cutting back comes with rewards. You get to rest and look after yourself and your loved ones. Minimalism adopts many methods. In clearing your closet, your schedule, or your storage room, the fact remains true that your entire lifestyle will benefit.

Tick the appropriate box for each remark

	Remark	Yes	Maybe	No
1	I have an overwhelming work schedule			
2	My health has been linked to my busy life			
3	I believe my physical well-being can improve if I cut down on some commitments			
4	My health stands in the way of my efficiency at work			

Earned Liberty

If utility is considered when it comes to the accumulation of quantifiable properties, one would be taken aback with the sudden realization of the primary motive of trying to acquire more.

Visualize the liberty one is bound to experience if he/she could perhaps let go of the undue burden to impress and do what is needed. This would even liberate more freedom to engage in other things, such as taking days off, traveling, or even starting one's own company and finally getting to do the things you like.

A person is bound to excel in his/her choice of venture, provided he/she isn't inundated with the fear of losing all possessions. Living with such concerns is living in bondage. True liberty is living without fear.

Tick the appropriate box for each remark

	Remark	Yes	Maybe	No
1	I feel bound whenever I get			

	consumed in chasing after possessions		
2	I nurse fears of actually losing all my assets		
3	Placing limitations and control over my desire and lifestyle can help me live a happier life		
4	I try to please my friend and family by my life choices		
5	I desire to travel, take a break and do what I love most		

Spare Time

Today, declining offers and opportunities as they come can be complicated. This happens for several reasons. The fast-paced life, limited offers, and economic pressures can force our hands into jumping on any opportunity that arises without necessarily giving it much thought.

Another reason is the dread of missing in action; the fear of the unknown- "what if I say no and thereby miss out on a great deal?" another phobia we struggle with is the fear of being bored. "What will we do if we don't take the gig?"

The truth is incredible opportunities will be there continually, they'll never be completely exhausted. Missing a couple doesn't spell doom; it only means you still have space for bigger and better ones coming ahead.

So, don't be afraid to clear your schedule in order to spend quality times with people and things that matter to you and yours. Host a cocktail, barbeque, or dinner with friends; go for walks and read another novel. Spend your time with what you cherish most; because time is a resource.

In many ways, not saying 'no' is a way of showing how self-focused you can be. It's like being obsessed with only you. By abandoning the old identity in that you chose minimalism, you begin to form a new character, a considerable part of which rotates around involvement in the lives of others. Paying attention beyond ourselves comes along with it a sense of satisfaction that we can't ever purchase at any store.

Tick the appropriate box for each remark

	REMARK	YES	MAYBE	NO
1	I feel saying 'no' can be dangerous for my career growth			
2	I think clearing my schedule will mean			

	saying 'no' to many offers		
3	I fear what losses I might incur once I say 'no.'		
4	I would love to spend quality time with friends and family		

Self- Assurance

It is possible to have complete self-assurance and self-confidence without amassing the most desirable properties or the latest pieces of fashion and trending items. The feeling can indeed be relieving and scintillating. This is at least one of the many benefits of living with less. You begin to feel good about yourself, not because of what you own but just because of who you are.

The entire lifestyle of a minimalist encourages independence and self-reliance, making you more poised in your quest of bliss. The inner strength to be able to surf life with nothing but sheer confidence in one's self must be awakened and sustained. This is non- negotiable, as it leads to various choices that can make or break effective practice of a minimalist lifestyle.

The desire to be known from and by the outward spillage must be thoroughly quenched and replaced with the fuzzy fling of being firmly rooted upon the grounds of self- reliance, self- worth and freedom from societal bondage.

Tick the appropriate box for each remark

	REMARK	YES	MAYBE	NO
1	I am a victim of societal pressure to conform			
2	My choices have primarily been influenced by the need to gain			

	acceptance			
3	I feel there is a connection between what I possess and how I should be seen by others			
4	Adopting a simple lifestyle will help relieve the pressure imposed by society			
5	I think it is possible to be happy and self-confident without actually associating it with any material thing			

Healthier connections

In the long run, when you feel you can quit competing with your associates and maybe your kinfolk to have the most elegant cars or the most massive dynasty; when you think you can stop attempting to amaze people and simply begin to bond with them on so many levels; when you feel you can let go of your trying-to-please-people tendencies and just go on to being yourself, it shouldn't come to you as some kind of shock when you notice that your relationships and connections begin to improve.

Also, great relationships are not put together on shady grounds, such as guilt or rivalry; they are instead built on collective effort and great memories.

Once you cease from trying to astonish others with your consumerist medals, you would be able to reposition your affairs by placing primary relations as fundamental, ancillary relationships as subsequent and marginal relationships as preceding.

Tick the appropriate box for each remark

	REMARK	YES	MAYBE	NO
1	My family and friends mean the world to me any			

	time, any day			
2	I feel associations that are founded on shady grounds always come back to haunt me			
3	Having a healthy relationship means not trying to please the people all the time			
4	Choosing a minimalist lifestyle will significantly help in improving every connection I have			

Generational Memories

The norm, especially during festive periods is to buy gifts and overspend on what isn't needed but an obligation to purchase, all in a bid to please and make good impressions to others and society. Fun memories are great substitutes for needless spending; you can initiate a fun road trip for instance, with your family; or a bush camp with friends. This might not be expensive to put together, but it will birth priceless memories.

When you take deliberate steps in migrating your focus from owning and buying stuff to building priceless memories, you probably may have a good store of memories to keep you smiling at the end of the day.

Memories, unlike gold and silver, are extremely priceless; can't be bought in any store. They are built over time and can serve as social platforms to rejuvenate the soul in dark times. Treasure them, and make as many as you can. Shifting your focus this way will equally help you remodel and reshape your outlook to life and its surroundings.

Tick the appropriate box for each remark

REMARK	YES	MAYBE	NO

1	I haven't deliberately invested in building up priceless memories		
2	I often have thought physical possessions can replace pleasant memories any day		
3	It is crucial to share fond memories with the people I love		
4	Living simply can help me make out time to hook up with friends and family		
5	Each encounter leaves something to be		

> remembered. I have to make each one count

More Cash

Purchasing less and being billed less would most definitely imply having a little bit of some extra cash on hand. This, of course, shouldn't come as a shocker to anyone. Indulging less and less in impulsive buying, surprise birthday parties, eating out, on-the- spot financial commitments all have to be nipped in the bud sooner, rather than later. This, of course, doesn't in any way imply that you spend your hard-earned cash on inferior goods. In fact, because of the level of discipline exhibited by an average minimalist, the purchasing of quality goods is not only possible but vital, as buying such quality goods would guarantee a longer lifespan; which also means that there would be no replacements for such purchases any time in the nearest future.

Saving up some extra money can be a motivating factor for most to embrace minimalism. Having more money and spending far less in a society that everyone is in debt can look like an impossibility, but it is possible. Minimalism upholds the norm that one's actual value isn't defined by his/her net worth but by self- worth.

Tick the appropriate box for each remark

	REMARK	YES	MAYBE	NO
1	I have the urge to spend heavily on items which I do not need.			
2	My appetite for luxury has bled my hard-earned revenue.			
3	I feel I can be happier if I redefine myself by my self- worth rather than by			

	my net worth.			
4	My financial choices can improve if I set my mind to spend wisely			
5	I can buy less and still buy smart; I can reduce quantity while still maintaining quality			

Chapter 11: 7 Step System To Minimalism And Decluttering Anything

This chapter is very important for you if you want to adopt minimalism and declutter your home.

Below, I will show you 7 detailed steps to follow:

Step #1: Start by taking inventory of everything you have

Put aside what is useful. For the rest, classify them into three categories:

Donate (If it is profitable)

Sell (If it has value)

Recycle (If it is broken and obsolete)

This is the most complicated part of starting to be a minimalist since many objects have a personal value for us or we are not ready for a radical discard. Take all the time you need, months or even years, for the process to be the most pleasant experience for you.

Would you get rid of 75% of your belongings?

How difficult is that? Do you know why?

Experts agree that there are two reasons:

☐ We are too clingy of the past

☐ We fear the near future

Gifts, memories, many things that you accumulate have great sentimental value. You can feel guilty just for thinking about throwing away that wonderful pink music box that your grandmother gave you when you were 9 years old. It is almost broken, yet you have kept it as a reminder of her or that precious time spent with her. How about the glass jar filled with sand from your first trip to the ocean, the collection of exchange cards, etc.

Are you really going to forget that person or will that memory be erased from your mind for not having "that object?" You have to get used to the idea that it is an object, yes, just that. Maintaining it will not make you go back to the past or relive that time. You have to realize that objects don't have feelings. It's you who is pouring the feeling and emotions into the objects. You will never be able to look to the future if your focus is in the past. The time has come to look forward and leave the past behind. What seems painful to you now, sometime later, you will wonder why you didn't do it before.

Step #2: Eliminate duplicates

Throughout process 1, you will find many useful things that you have to keep, but of which you will soon find that can have a high amount of. An example is over a dozen cups, five boxes of silverware, many towels and tablecloths, etc. If they are in a poor condition, recycle them. Whatever is in an average state, start using. Items that are in a very good condition keep it in boxes so that it does not occupy so much space.

The box: just in case

There is a trick on the Internet that everyone says works very well. Have a box for "just in case" things. These are items where your internal dialogue is, "What if I need it."

There is only one rule for the box.

After one year, if you have not used it, remove it from your home. You don't need it. That will be your way of seeing what you really need and what is only occupying space in your life.

The 3 questions you should ask each time you doubt

Every time you start to doubt whether to save something or not, ask yourself these three questions:

When did you use it for the last time?

And this comes to the thread of the previous trick, the one with the "just in case" box. When was the last time you put on those pants? When was the last time you used the exercise bike? Has it become the coat rack in the room? Are you really going to put on that lipstick again? And what about the 50 notebooks and washi-tapes you have started using or the ones still in their plastic packaging?

If you have not used that object for more than a year (if you remember that it existed), take it out. You don't need it

Is it in good condition?

It's broken? Is it missing any piece? Has the paint vanished? Does it have a stubborn stain ? If you can think of a solution and are sure you will be able to fix it, set a date and time to fix it. If not, you know the drill, take it outside.

If in a year you have not fixed it, you now know, you really do not have a use for it in your home, and it is just cluttering up space.

Is it something useful or is it an ornament?

Is it outdated? Do you have too many of it? Is it something that makes life easier for you, saves and makes you money or time? Maybe, if you got rid of it, you could buy that other ornament that is in trend now or buy the newest model that has the functions you need right now.

Yes, you can give the item another chance but set a time limit. If you have not utilised the item or do not have the same sentimental feelings about it, it is best to remove it from your life.

Step #3: Declare areas free of junk

Always propose to leave certain areas free of junk, such as the kitchen countertop, your study desk (It's okay to leave a notepad and a plant), your bedside table, and propose not to fill them with anything that wasn't strictly necessary and useful in that space. In that way, you avoid accumulating and acquiring new objects for those surfaces.

How do you perform a minimalist cleaning?

Let's start step by step. Choose a room, and from there you will expand the cleaning to the rest of the rooms until you have cleaned the whole home. From the chosen room, establish the order of "sites" to be cleaned. You can start with the drawer on the table. If it's something traumatic for you, you can stop there the first day and move to the next table the next day. From there to the first drawer of the wardrobe, another day the second, and before you know it, you have finished the first room. You can also set a cleaning order and set a time to do it every day; 15 minutes, 30 minutes. You choose what works best for you. The only rule is to fulfill the plan that you are going to establish.

Necessary material

The base of success is good planning. So, before you start cleaning, make sure you have the following in hand:

A large garbage bag, the garden type variety ones. Keep several handy because you will certainly need a few.

3 boxes in which you will classify each object as follows:

One for the things that stay.

Another for the things that go.

And another for the things you doubt.

Post-it of colors: In case you have something in volume or too many things to classify, and you want to advance in a quicker way. Each post-it color represents a destination; it stays, it goes away, I have doubts.

Cleaning materials: It is best to take advantage of it and every time you have an "empty space" (drawer, shelf ...) take advantage of it by removing the dust, wiping the insides with a damp cloth and then drying with a dry cloth.

Step #4: Start traveling light

Warning: This is not a tutorial on how to fold and hide clothes in bags; this is a tutorial to take as little as possible, the only REAL way to save space in the suitcase.

Reducing the number of things you pack for travel will help you realize what you really need. Soon you will discover that if you spend 4 days out, you will only need to take clothes for 2 days if you wash your clothes by hand during the trip (which in turn will make you realize that even in your own home you don't need as many clothes as you thought before). Beginning to be a minimalist in travel will help you in your daily life, helping you reduce the number of things you always had on you.

Step #5: Be clear about how much your time is worth

Just as we are addicted to spending money, so are we to spend time. An essential part of minimalism is to reconnect with you and your needs, which also applies to your time. Your time is limited, and that is why you must learn to say no and to structure it around what really matters. The first step is to know how much your time is really worth.

A trick that can help you is to measure the price in working hours.

How to put it into practice?

You were very clear that you wanted a mobile phone to use and yet shortly after entering the store you were looking at the mid-high range because they looked better. In the end, you ended up with a state-of-the-art device in your pocket. 536 Euros, no more no less

How is it possible?

Stores use many tricks to sell more without you noticing they are exploiting vulnerabilities of human psychology. On the other, your own brain plays against you when it comes to buying. It's what behavioral economics calls behavioral biases. Here you can see the traps that you are most likely to fall into. A good example is the traps of 0% financing offers. The result, in any case, is you will buy more than what you were actually planning to spend on.

The solution is to apply a simple trick; the method of calculating the price in working hours.

How the method of measuring your purchases during working hours works?

Start measuring what you buy according to the hours you will have to work to achieve it is a tool that works for two reasons.

Reason 1

It prevents you from making impulsive decisions. Instead of buying what you want directly, you will have to stop for a few seconds to think about how many hours of work the mobile phone or television you want costs you. Even if you have to take out your mobile to use the calculator, those seconds will stop your consumer craving.

Reason 2

Knowing how many hours of work means buying something will help you better identify your priorities. You will have a more realistic perspective of what things cost you and what you must 'suffer' to achieve them.

How to calculate the price in working hours?

Do you want to know how much an hour of your work is worth? This is what you must do to calculate how much your work is worth an hour and be able to make financial decisions.

Process #1: Have the following data on hand; your annual gross salary and the number of hours you work per year.

Process #2: Divide the salary by the number of hours worked.

Process #3: Enter this figure and keep it in mind to make purchasing decisions, so that it helps you control what you buy and you will not buy more.

Step # 6: Enter one, one goes out

Once you have managed to reduce all your unnecessary things you can follow this principle; if something comes into your life, something has to go out. For example, would you buy a new golf set if the one you have is only six months old and you are the only golf player in your home? If you follow this principle, the answer would be no. If you decide to go ahead, then if something goes in, something comes out. (In this case, the six-month-old golf set).

This is something you commit yourself to. If you do not comply, you're only hurting yourself. The moment you break your commitment to this principle, the effort of having to solve the problem of accumulating useless things grows.

Yes, I agree. It is complicated to apply, very difficult for people like you and me.

But in the end, even if it's just for economic reasons, it makes you think whether it's really worth accepting that gift or spending your money on something you already have and not taking advantage of it as you should.

Step #7: Consider making a big change

Moving to a smaller space is not for everyone. However, if you rent and the price is increasing or if you really have problems paying at the end of the month, reducing the space will help you in several ways; to have fewer things, to spend less time cleaning and, of course, to spend less.

Do it with intelligence, avoid comparisons. Your minimalism belongs only to you. It is what works for you, in your life, and at this moment. If you want to keep each book you read but only have 12 items in your closet, then do it.

Chapter 12: Possessions: Less Is More

After you've gone through the steps of getting the right mindset as described in chapter two, now comes practical application. It's one thing to think that you need to cut back, it's another to actually do it. You have to cross this threshold. For minimalism to work for you and become part of your daily living experience, you have to act on it.

The good news is cutting up possessions is actually easier than you think. Seriously. Why?

Well, just look at the contents of your desk. Pay attention to your bookshelf. Take a look around your room. You will realize that there's a lot of clutter. There is a lot of stuff there that doesn't absolutely need to be there. Now, with that said, there's always a hierarchy.

There are things that are like low-hanging fruit. These are the things that you can obviously cut out. Unfortunately, once you clear that away, your job isn't done. There are a lot of things that you think you can't go without but are actually expendable.

So, it's really important to have some sort of game plan coming in. You can't just do things by the seat of your pants, and let your emotions and impulses drive you as to which parts to cut out. That's not going to work.

Chances are, you might be sorry for the stuff you let go and agonize about stuff that you know you need to let go, but you feel you can't. So, you remain stuck. And if you stay stuck for a long enough period of time, you give up.

I don't want that to happen to you, so I want you to come into that situation with some sort of advance plan. Again, this whole book is a framework. It's not a set of rules, so here are just some suggestions.

Start as Close to Home as Possible

Where is your home? No, it's not the four corners of the place you're living in. Your home is your mind. Your home is the place in the universe from which you observe and interact with the rest of the universe. Start as close to your home as possible.

So, this means shrinking your circle of focus. As far as your day to day body goes, what can you let go? So, you start with your clothes. You start with your eyewear. You start with your footwear. I could go on and on.

The key to this is to shrink your circle of focus. Right now, you're reading this book and you're looking around you, and you're overwhelmed. I get that. I understand fully where you're coming from. The reason why you're overwhelmed is because your circle of focus is too broad. It's too wide. You're just taking in so much at one time.

Shrink your circle of focus as close to your mind and body as possible.

Now, look at your closet. Look at your shoe rack. Pay attention to the accessories on your desk. Look at your desk. Next, apply the framework that you arrived at from chapter two. Which of these things do you need? Which of these things take so much maintenance and worry, that it overwhelms you? Again, only you know the answer.

Similarly, focus on your circle of control. At this point, focus on the things that you can immediately let go. What can you control right now? This is crucial because a lot of the stuff that you own is actually owned by somebody else.

Maybe you're living with your girlfriend or boyfriend, or you have a husband or wife. You can't just chuck stuff out because they own that as well. Similarly, you may owe stuff to the bank, or you may be paying stuff off.

If you paid for stuff with a credit card, you can chuck that. But if you are still paying to the bank in the form of a mortgage or amortization, you might want to slow down and look at other options. I'm not saying you should not get rid of it. I'm saying that you should look at reselling.

So, for example, if you live in a home and you quickly realize that you really only need maybe 30 square meters or 300 square feet, but you live in a home that is 1,200 square feet or even more. What do you do then? After all, it's not paid off yet. You're still making monthly payments to the bank. Start planning to sell your home. Start looking up realtors.

Regardless, focus on your circle of control. These are the things that you can directly control, and from there, radiate out to the things that you share control with or that you owe money on.

Proactive versus Reactive

It's crucial that you be proactive as much as possible when letting go of possessions. The problem is, a lot of people are reactive. They just look at the things around them and basically only choose to let go of the stuff that is screaming to be let go.

For example, if you have a velvet Elvis painting that you bought on a whim, it's easy to chuck that. That's screaming to be let go regardless of your taste in art. But you have to go beyond that.

You have to be proactive and really apply the analysis that I've walked you through in chapter two to all the items in your surroundings. Otherwise, it's very easy to come up with some sort of justification at some level or another why you need to hang on to these things.

You end up in the same place. You'll end up in square one. So be proactive as much as possible.

Cutting Back Means More Control

I know a part of you is struggling as you put that item in the moving box so you can sell it off or give it away. There's a struggle going on inside you. Believe me, I understand. I've been there. But also focus on the fact that when you cut back and you let go, it means more control, so whatever is left over is easier to manage.

The value of the things that are leftover is more obvious to you. You're not bargaining with yourself. You're not coming up with some sort of excuse or explanation or justification. Instead, it's obvious that you need whatever is left over, and this is control.

You can probably say to yourself everything that I can see around me is exactly what I need. Think about that for a second. Few people can say that. Few people can even realize that. Do you see how much control you have? So, dwell on this as you struggle putting stuff in the box.

Cutting Back Means More Accountability

In addition to control over the remainders, please understand that you become more accountable to yourself when you cut back. Here's the problem: when we surround ourselves with possessions, it's easy to lose ourselves in our possessions.

It's easy to trick ourselves into thinking that we need everything, and that's why the credit card bills that keep piling up are absolutely justified. Now, stop playing games with yourself. What you've done is the precise opposite. What you've managed to achieve is you have let go of all sense of accountability.

You're not being responsible. You're throwing good money after bad and you're just basically chasing this illusionary tie or association between material things and what you truly are looking for, a sense of emotional payoff, and the more you do this, the less accountable you become to yourself or anybody else. This is irresponsible living.

I know that this is all harshly phrased, and I did that for a specific reason. I want it to burn because it is only when it burned and it stung that I was able to wake up to this fact when I first practiced minimalism. You should do the same.

Cutting back means more accountability to yourself and to others. By letting go of the financial drain as well as the financial obligations to those things, you have a lot more to share those who need your help.

Cutting Back Means Less Clutter

Sorry if this comes off as so obvious that it almost doesn't need to be said, but you have to understand that clutter operates on many different levels. The most obvious clutter, of course, is the one that you can see. This is the type of clutter that make you feel squeezed, pressured, limited, stressed, and all sorts of negative mental and emotional states.

Obviously, if you put stuff in a box, there's less of that, but there's also emotional clutter. You're worried less about stuff that may get lost, stolen, damaged, corrupted, degraded, fermented, I can go on and on.

To make things clear and to give you the emotional and intellectual drive you need to get out from under clutter, I want you to wrap your mind around the key concept of return on investment.

Now, you may be thinking to yourself, what does ROI have to do with minimalism? After all, ROI is usually about finances, and minimalism if anything involves an attitude that tries to free itself from the toxic effects of finances. So, what am I talking about?

Well, everything that you buy has a cost and a benefit. You buy things because you're after those benefits. You're looking for a return. The money that you pay is your investment. Everything has an ROI.

And when you decide to cut back on clutter, you have to come to the realization, and I'm not talking about you just taking my word for it. I'm talking about you reading my words and fully understanding it, and agreeing that it applies to your life. You have to make sense of this. If it doesn't make sense right now, go back to chapter two.

If you come to the realization that much of your possessions no longer deliver a solid ROI, then it becomes easier to cut back on clutter. At this point, you have gone from thinking of things in terms of physical clutter to emotional and mental clutter.

Ask yourself, that trinket that you bought on the trip to the grocery store, is it still delivering the kind of emotional buzz that you were searching for? Do this with all the other stuff that you picked up along the way. You should be able to see a pattern.

Wouldn't you want to get off that treadmill of initial buzz, anticipation, excitement and then ultimately not even caring? It gets old, right? The problem is, your finances spiral out of control. Even worse, you feed an addiction. You see the pattern. You see the dopamine burst at first, so you repeat it over and over again. Dopamine, serotonin, all those other "happy chemical" neurotransmitters in your brain.

It's spiraling out of control. The more you do this, the stronger the addiction holds. So, the key is to break out of that, and this is where your personal psychology steps in. You want to break out of that spiral. There's the emotional angle, as well as the physical and material outcome. But the psychological aspect is also important.

You ought to put your foot down. Try to say that this is a dead-end, it just gets worse and worse. Before you know it, this becomes a personal, moral and philosophical issue. You start living for things, and your self-esteem is defined by how you look in front of other people instead of values you chose for yourself, as well as your genuine care for other people, and this all leads to a lack of control on so many levels.

So, cut back on the physical clutter and allow it to trigger you cutting back on other forms of clutter. Mental, emotional and psychological.

Start Now

This is where the rubber meets the road. That part is obvious. Unfortunately, a lot of people are experts at tricking themselves into waiting for tomorrow. They keep saying to themselves, "Not now. I know what I need to do. I know the right thing to do. I get all of that and I 100% agree. I realize all of that and I'm ready to do it tomorrow."

Here's the problem. Tomorrow never comes. Life, after all, is what happens when you're making other plans. You will find a way to distract yourself from doing what you need to do, so it happens. You keep kicking the can down the road, and tomorrow never comes.

Stop playing this game with yourself. You have to cut, and you have to cut now and cut clean.

Cut and Track

Keep track of what you cut. So, when you're putting stuff in that moving box, keep an inventory sheet. What exactly are you letting go of? When you start with your body, get on a schedule. Say to yourself, "Okay, for this week I'm going to be cutting back on personal care items. Then for next week, I'll be cutting back on clothing," so on and so forth.

Not only are you able to cut but you're able to maintain letting go because there is some sort of objective measure or tracking system. You're not just doing things at the seat of your pants or out some sense of emotional urgency that may be here today and completely gone tomorrow.

This is crucial. Start close to home. So, start with your mind, then your body, then work outwards from there. This can mean the desk that you constantly sit in front of every single day, so empty out the drawers, go through the items and chuck what you can get rid of. Once you're done with that, look over to your bookshelf and repeat the process.

At the end of this process, you would have started from your inner core all the way to your closet, your file drawers, your desk drawers, your bookshelf, and even your kitchen pantry and garage. Start within and work outwards.

Chapter 13: By Choosing To Be A Minimalist, You Will Be More Productive

Have you ever thought about how many things which you own you don't even use or don't even know the purpose of? Does this realization make you more stressed?

Now let's imagine the opposite situation: You are completely aware of all of your possessions and you can very quickly remember all the things that you own and the reason for owning those things. Doesn't this second situation feel so much better? This approach will actually provide you with a lot more energy and a lot less stress and your productivity will skyrocket as a result. This may be subtle, but the chances are high that the mess and the lack of organization in your home impact your productivity in a negative way.

If you want to be able to do good work, then you have to make sure that you intentionally design your working space. This doesn't have to be complicated since complexity is the enemy of execution. For example, when your home is more pleasant, then you will be more likely to stick to your hygienic habits and your other healthy habits that have to get done.

When you have to search every corner and every drawer to find what you want, that adds up over the course of days and weeks and you can lose a lot of your time and energy which will ensure that your life will take a hit. This chapter is all about showing you how being more minimalistic can improve your productivity with your work and all areas of life.

Design Your Home Office

When most people think about being productive at home, they will think of something like a personal office within their homes where they keep all necessary things for doing the work such as a computer or relevant files and all the other items that may be helpful. It is necessary to plan and to know what may be necessary for the work so that you don't get interrupted by having to look for things that aren't within the reach of your hand.

If you are fortunate enough to have a career which allows you to work from home, or if you just like to have space within your home where you do your administrative duties, then this chapter will prove to be quite helpful.

For the most people, this office space within a home will not be very tidy and organized and it will look like a bomb went off when you see all the papers and tools and cables lying around.

In order to get this organized, you need to make sure that you have a system for organizing your documents. The good old filing cabinet will do the trick here. You do have to know which documents are actually appropriate for filling since there are some documents which you may need to use more frequently. You can achieve this kind of organization by using paper trays and you should use those while keeping how human memory works in mind.

You should have one tray which is used for all the current projects which are handled right at the moment of working. This tray should be dealt with every day and it is necessary to get rid of things that shouldn't be there anymore by either getting rid of them or putting them on another tray.

At the end of the work week, which will most likely be Friday, you will take anything that is still left on the current tray and you will place it in the filing cabinet if you deem it important enough while throwing away anything else that is considered unimportant. This is effective because it is acknowledged that there are some things that may require quick access and recovery. Also, by sticking to this system over the course of time, you make sure that the paperwork doesn't pile up and that it is put where it won't be able to create a mess.

If you can, then you should make an effort to reduce the quantity of paper you are working with. You should always have some kind of notepad with you so that you could capture ideas before they disappear and you should always think if converting a certain document to a digital format makes sense and you should do so if you determine that digitalization is the best choice.

By doing this, the organization will be so much easier. It is also a good idea to invest in a scanner which you can use to scan important documents so that you could convert them into a file that will be possible to work with on a computer. If you think that a physical form of the scanned document is no longer necessary, then you can simply get rid of it.

If you implement these changes into your system, the work which is required for paperwork all around your home will be much easier to manage and that will ensure that your home makes it easier for you to be productive.

Again, knowing how to manage your cables is pretty important. If it is possible to use a wireless variant for certain electronics, then you should do so since it will make your life so much easier. If you are really serious about this, then you can purchase a product such as Amazon Echo which will allow you to issue voice commands to your computer.

In order to be more productive, it is all about making the procedures simpler and removing the obstacles and doing this fairly regularly. The fewer steps there are to completing a certain task, the more efficient a system is. Everything that you may require to do your work should be within your reach and this is a variant of French cooking concept known as mise en place. Designing your home like this will save you hours.

The goal of removing clutter and obstacles is to make getting the work done easier and smoother. If a certain item or a certain piece of furniture doesn't serve a purpose within your office, then you should get rid of it from your office to make things easier for you. Any extra items that are in your office have the potential to be a distraction and that is why you should carefully consider what is in your office and what isn't. You want to make a separation between your working life and your personal life and doing this actually resets your brain.

The place in which the work is done shouldn't be used to do fun things and that is why a bookshelf or a TV has no reason for being there since that will only put ideas of fun in your head. The room in which you do your work shouldn't necessarily be bland and it is actually a good idea to add some color to that room if that will help your productivity. When choosing a color, remember that certain colors are better for productivity instead of others and light green, for example, is relaxing since it is similar to what you would see when looking at plants and that simply feels good.

The point is that if you don't like corporate looking environments, then you shouldn't design your working space as one. Just make sure that the room in which you do work doesn't have things which have the potential to distract you and this will make procrastination a whole lot harder. Using each line of defense against procrastination is necessary.

Make Sure That Your Electronics Remain Clean and Fast

It is important for a piece of technology to keep doing its job well and without hiccups. Just as you want to make sure that the room in which you are doing your work is nice and tidy and without clutter, you want to apply the same logic and the same rules to the computer you are working on. If the desktop of your computer is covered with icons that you don't use, then that is also an issue for productivity since that will stress you out. That could also slow down your computer and that will also cause a lot of stress which will ruin your productivity plans.

You want to take the organization of your files seriously since you don't want for important files to go missing. You also don't want for your computer to be too slow since that will make you anxious each and every time you boot up your computer. The minimalistic design principles are not limited to only your room and you should be applying them to the design of your computer as well. If there is an unnecessary file, then you want , and you also want to make sure that your antivirus software is a good one. You also want to know if there is a good reason for installing a particular piece of software. It is extremely satisfying when your computer is running as it should and when you are not being taken out of the flow of the work by a slow computer.

Chapter 14: Experiencing Life More Means Overcoming Convenience Addiction

One of the most damaging fictions that we can believe in is the cult of comfort and convenience. We're not entitled to a comfortable and convenient life. We're entitled to having a chance. Often times, we have to make our way to get that shot, but we're definitely not entitled to results.

Unfortunately, that's the kind of mindset too many people have. It holds them back and drags them down. The bottom line is a lot of the things that we're unhappy about as a culture are due to our addiction to convenience.

Weight Problems

In study after study, public health institutions and research groups agree that Americans as a group are getting fatter and slower with time. Other studies suggest that Americans are also getting unhappier over time. These are all interrelated because we are devoted to convenience. In fact, our devotion is almost slavish. We can't get enough convenience.

The problem is what you do with the time you spend. You sit in front of the computer, or a screen. You spend countless hours in front of a tablet instead of walking around or engaging in some kind of physical activity, we take the time that has been freed up by our time-saving devices to lead almost effort-free lives. That's why we're getting fatter and fatter, slower and slower, and more miserable.

This is quite a paradox, but if you think about it, modern Western society is a victim of its own success. Why do you think anti-anxiety and antidepressant medications are always in the top ten most prescribed drugs in the United States? They go hand in hand. It seems that the more convenient life becomes, the more unhappy people become.

How to Break Free

In this chapter, I'm going to help you break free from your addiction to convenience. Is it going to be easy? Absolutely not. Are you going to have a good time? Of course not. Is it absolutely necessary? You bet so.

What is the first thing that you need to do? First, do things the hard way. Instead of taking that elevator, try to take one flight of stairs up. That's all I ask, one flight of stairs. It's not going to kill you, so try it. Instead of parking at that reserve spot right next to the entrance to your office, or the nearest entrance to the shopping mall, park at the farthest parking spot, and walk all the way.

This is pretty basic. At first, it's going to be annoying. I can grant you that, but the more you do this, the more it becomes second nature. You may be the type of person who has a tough time getting up in the morning and running a few laps around your block, but when you resolve to do things the hard way, even minor inconveniences like parking really far away can make you adopt a more physically active lifestyle in a totally passive way.

As long as you don't think about it, and you just make it part of your daily routine, you're actually increasing the amount of activity you do every single day. This makes things more inconvenient, but your mind adapts. It turns out that you didn't really need to park right next to the entrance, or you can wait an hour or thirty minutes for pizza, and that extra fifteen or forty five minutes is not going to kill you. Who knew, right?

Do things the hard way. Break that shell of convenience addiction ever so slightly. The good news is the moment cracks start to appear, is when you can start scaling it up. Your world did not fall apart. You did not die. You're still there, and you can take some more inconvenience.

Practical Tip: Walk More

Not only should you walk to your office or a farther distance at school, try to walk more. Even if you work as a freelancer, and you're basically writing or dictating stuff all day, make it a point to get up and walk for about ten minutes every hour.

It's not going to kill you. In fact, according to research studies, sitting down for extended periods of time is a good indicator that you might die earlier than anticipated. However, walking more also primes your mind. You're not just diving into stuff that's quick and easy by walking around more, but you're also more physically active and take stock of what's around you. You gain a greater appreciation of what you have around you as well.

Practical Tip: Take Your Time

Allow yourself to wait more. If you ever find yourself in a line, don't get upset. I know a lot of Americans really blow a fuse when they have to wait for longer than thirty minutes.

Redeem the time by whipping out a pocket book and start reading. You're actually doing two things at that point. You're multitasking. Not only are you adding value to your intellectual powers by reading, but you're also waiting in lines, so you're going to be there for your appointment. It's going to pan out. You just have to wait.

The Big Payoff

These things may seem small, but let me tell you; they pay off really well. First of all, you develop greater discipline. I'm sure you don't need me to tell you how important discipline is.

Discipline is all about doing things that are necessary when you have other easier and more convenient things you can do. You put in the hard work now, so you can get a bigger reward in the future. Doing the easy stuff now, on the other hand, yields to lower level rewards or lower quality rewards.

Adding more inconvenient activities to your day also results in greater patience. You are able to put up with a lot more stuff from other people. You are also able to put in time in otherwise trying situations. Let's face it; it's human nature to take the path of least resistance.

Instead of having to wait for a significant other or a family member to get his or her act together, it's so much easier just to hit the exit. Who needs the inconvenience or hassle, right? If you want your relationships to blossom, you have to be there and hang in there.

All these pay off on a mental level. You get to enjoy the process, see life play out and see more details. These details are what actually count. Do you think life is a race where you get extra points for soaking up as many "good things in life" as you make your way from point A to Point B? Probably not.

The person who dies after stopping to smell the roses probably has a lot more happier memories than somebody who's just on this mad dash to accumulate everything and experience everything. At the end of the day, it's probably just a bucket list. So what? Enjoy the process and see how life plays out in all its beauty and ugliness. That's what life is. It's a mix. Get over it or embrace it.

Chapter 15: Ways You Can Embrace Minimalism Every Day

This chapter will look at simple ways in which you can embrace Minimalism every day, no matter where you are or what you are doing.

The great thing about being a minimalist is there is no right or wrong way of doing it. You can start small, such as having a minimalist approach to your:

- Interior design
- Clothes
- Makeup, or
- Traveling in the simplest means possible.

You can apply it to just one area of your life or you can embrace Minimalism in every aspect of your day.

Shopping

Just because you are a minimalist, that doesn't mean you can't go shopping anymore. Not at all – we all genuinely need new things sometimes. Rather than giving up shopping all together and bracing yourself for the next year of using the same clothes, towels, and bed linen until they go to dust, Minimalism encourages you to be conscious when you are shopping and make careful, deliberate choices. When you go to the supermarket, take a list with you of everything you need and just buy those items. I know it's often all too tempting when you see a promotion that is such a bargain that it would be a crime to leave it, but this is the consumer culture at work again. Stick to your list and when you get home, you probably will have forgotten that amazing promotion anyway.

Start Saying 'No'

Minimalism isn't all about having a material-free place. It's about you leading the life you want without distractions. One of the most important things we could all learn is how to say 'no' to things we don't want to do. It's all too easy to say yes to your boss when he asks you to work overtime when you don't want to, or to agree to go out for dinner with your friends when you're tired and just want to stay at home, especially if you are a people-pleaser. One of the main reasons we do this is because we are worried how the other person will react – maybe they will be upset, offended or even get angry. However, the reality is they probably won't mind at all and at the end of the day, you are not responsible for how they react to your 'no'. Next time someone asks you to go out with them and you don't want to, try saying 'no' and concentrate on doing what you truly want to do.

Experiences, Not Things

Start making this your mantra if it helps – experiences over things. Rather than buying material items, think of the experiences you could have instead and the memories you can create. For example, if you already have a perfectly decent TV at home, why buy the newest, more expensive one? Just think of:

- where you could travel to

- what a lovely meal you could have at the fanciest restaurant, or

- how relaxed you will feel after a day at the spa.

Swap your material items for memories and happiness.

Minimalism with Internet

So, you work on the computer, and rather than finishing your report or updating your customer's details, you find yourself browsing through the most obscure information on Wikipedia or Quora, wondering how you ended up there. Or, you are waiting for the bus, and rather than appreciating the drama of the rainclouds or reflections in the puddles, you are aimlessly scrolling down Instagram looking at photos of people you haven't seen in years. Maybe that sounds a little dramatic, but it is so easy to get sucked into the digital world and miss what's going on around us.

Try browsing with intention, and only when you specifically need something. When you are looking for something to do, enjoy the scenery, read a book, or listen to music. This simple act helps you to live more in the moment, and appreciate the little things in life that can be immensely rewarding.

Chapter 16: Minimalism And Discipline

One thing that I've noticed throughout my life is that proper and true minimalists are very well disciplined — which can be considered as a benchmark. Just because you've decided to become a minimalist and have reduced some clutter from your surroundings doesn't make you a minimalist. Minimalism is a lifestyle that takes painstaking efforts (mostly psychological) day-by-day effort to integrate into your life. Take military personnel from any corner of the globe as a prime example. These men and women can survive in harsh conditions that would give most of us common folk the jitters with the bare minimum that can be fit into a 40-pound rucksack, truly living up to George Clooney's famous minimalist backpacker monologue from the critically acclaimed film Up In The Air. So how does the average Joe or Jane turn into such amazing minimalists within a matter of 2-3 years of training and overcome their previous lifestyle and mindset? No matter which walk of life they come from, or what race or religion they belong to, armies all around the world embrace everyone. By the time they're done training, all these men and women possess some universal traits, one of which is minimalism. This minimalism is achieved by rigorous and stringent disciplined thinking and lifestyle, which brings out and engages a person to be the most efficient and effective versions of themselves. Make no mistake, before the military personnel is trained into soldiers, they're just regular people like you and me. In all probability, they used to watch the same T.V shows that we watch, liked hanging out at bars and pubs with friends, and enjoyed the same frivolities in life most people do. Despite all the hardships that they must go through during training, ask any military personnel you come across, and they'll tell you that life has become better for them thanks to discipline.

To be disciplined, one must be very focused on what they are doing. To be focused one needs to be a realist. As I discussed earlier, minimalism is the end of fantasies. To end your fantasies, you need to discipline. The first step to walking away from fantasies is letting go of the sources that fuel those fantasies, which can be anything depending on an individual's situation. It might sound like a natural thing when you're reading it, but unless you've tried it out yourself, you won't understand how difficult this task can be. Fantasies are like drugs, so getting rid of them can be quite tricky.

Discipline is the ability to control the base urges of the mind and body. As adults, the three basic things that most of us should be able to manage after years of education and experience are health, finances, and our possessions. Sadly, however, most of us fail to do so because of our desire for excess and failure to prioritize on the correct actions and decisions. This is because most people who are not minimalists are not disciplined enough to distinguish between what we need and what we want. I've seen countless people lamenting about their nine-to-five jobs and wishing they could start their own trade or practice but are unable to do so due to their lack of discipline. Even if you have a comfortable job with healthy income, don't spend money on unnecessary stuff. Having more money doesn't prevent you from being a minimalist, spending it unnecessarily does. Do you really need that new iPhone or those new Colin Kaepernick sneakers from Nike when you have a perfectly functioning phone or a decent pair of snickers? I'm sure deep inside you'll find that the answer is no.

The first step towards discipline and minimalism is to be aware of one's reasons and actions. Many people are not even aware of neither rhyme or reason for their actions. For example, a lot of people tend to walk into a fast-food joint with a bunch of friends, order a lot of food and leave significant amounts of leftovers once they're done with their meals which cannot be given away or recycled. These people don't prioritize their orders on how hungry they are, but rather on how many people have come for dinner, which is illogical and impractical when you think about it. When one becomes aware of why they're doing something, and what they're doing they start taking the first step toward minimalism and by effect, discipline.

One of the biggest reasons society and individuals are so undisciplined in the west is because they were not raised with the notion of self-accountability. Instead, western society emphasizes accountability to others. By my estimate, this is one of the biggest reasons why minimalism never found its proper place in the western culture, unlike its Eastern counterpart. Without self-accountability, one cannot truly understand what they need to prioritize to live a happy and fulfilling life. Most people stake their happiness on the opinion of society which measures a person's worth on how much they have instead of how much a person is contributing to social growth. Thus, we thrive on a culture of excess from the moment we step into the world. Even our personal standards are warped by a lack of self-accountability, not just our tendencies and habits. Assuming you've had a healthy romantic life and have dated a few people, think back on how your romantic preferences have changed over the years and from partner to partner. Most people look for exciting and superfluous qualities in a romantic partner in their younger years, trading out for a stable and dependable partner in their later years. Even if you're not a minimalistic person, you can clearly see that our romantic preferences become minimalistic as we age. This happens because our life partners are something that we are accountable for unlike many other things in life.

It's a give-and-take type of relationship on both ends. Discipline fuels minimalism by making the minimalist confident in their decisions and actions. One of the prime reasons we keep doing and buying things that we don't need is to confirm our self-validation through the approval of people around us. Once an individual finds their self-confidence and self-worth, they don't feel the urge to fit in with the crowd. When we can clearly define what we want through disciplined thinking and reflection, we learn to identify what's best for us and how to achieve it in the most straightforward manner. This is what happens to military personnel once they're done with training. The rose-tinted glasses of excess and indulgence they wore before joining the military falls off once they learn to think and evaluate everything in a practical manner. One of the biggest reasons Eastern societies have achieved minimalism successfully as a whole is because they're raised with discipline from birth. If children are given whatever they want, it sets them on an 'I want more' line of thinking which is very prevalent in many first world countries around the world.

The bottom line here is, minimalism and discipline are dependent on one another in such a way that you cannot master one without mastering the other.

Chapter 17: Minimalist Wardrobe

Do you know how many pairs of pants you own? How many shoes do you have? How many pairs of underwear do you have? What about socks? Do you have formal wear, casual work wear, and lazy days clothing?

How much is really enough when it comes to clothing? Minimalists believe you do not need a lot of clothing to look great. Instead, it is about how you pair your clothing to create different looks. There are several benefits to a minimalist wardrobe.

You save on closet space.

You do not have that much to wash, so you save on laundry expenses.

Your home is less cluttered.

You get rid of clothing that is no longer in great shape or that does not fit you.

You may have one of those closets that never feels like enough. You are constantly jamming clothing into your closet and ten pieces fall out when you try to remove one. This is a sign that you are hoarding clothing. Your closet is probably the perfect size, but you have excess clothing that is cluttering it.

What would happen if you only had two loads of laundry—one for clothing and one for towels/linens? Would you have more time and feel freer? Of course, you would. When you do not have to spend an entire day just on laundry, life becomes better. You have more of your days off to spend how you want to.

So, let's get there. What can you do to your wardrobe to have a "minimalist" closet?

Open your closet doors—don't faint from the sight!

Pull out one item. Does this item have holes? Is the color faded? Is there something about the item that is uncomfortable?

If you answered "no" to all three questions, you can place that clothing item in an area of your room that is designated the "keep" pile. If you answered "yes" to at least one of the questions it must leave your home.

Some items can be donated and others are simply rags that need to go in the trash. You will make the decision. If you saw the item at the thrift store would you buy it? If the answer is no, it goes in the trash.

You are going to go through your entire closet using the three-step assessment. If you are honest about the clothing you own, you should have a larger donate/trash pile than a keep pile.

You might eliminate clothing because it does not fit right, you no longer like the color or the pattern. When you assess clothing with a critical eye and not sentiment, it is easier to get rid of your excess clothing.

It is possible you could downsize even more on your wardrobe. Remove the items you do not want anymore, before proceeding.

Hang up the clothing you have kept. If not everything is going to be hung in your closet that is okay. Ultimately, what you want is to assess what you have and determine if you have multiple items in the same color and if you can keep two or three items instead of all of them.

Let's say you have five pairs of black dress pants and three black skirts. You have eight items to wear on your bottom. There are seven days in the week. You also have five pairs of jeans and two pairs of yoga pants. This is excessive since there are only seven days a week. You probably work three to five days a week, depending on your career choice.

You need at least three bottoms to wear during the week, and pants to wear on the weekend. If you choose wisely, your work wear can include three bottoms, with five different shirts.

If you do not want to go entirely minimalistic with your wardrobe, then keep a pair of pants, skirts, or dresses, for each day of the week. If you exercise three times a week, keep three workout outfits.

You do not have to have a wardrobe that offers 20 choices. You can have one that is enough for an entire week, with a couple of formal pieces for special occasions. One black dress or suit for dates is enough because you can use different accessories, such as scarves, ties, belts, and shoes to make the outfit appear different. You can also use work clothing as date clothing.

Buying New Clothes

If your wardrobe is ten years old, you might need new clothes. If you bought a piece here and there to wear, but overall your clothing is old, buy new items. You could take everything in your closet out. Sell what is in great shape, donate decent clothing, and trash the rest. Now, you start with new things.

You will always want to buy an item and get rid of an item if you are a minimalist. This works for anything—really. If you buy something, the rule is—you must get rid of something.

If you buy a new pair of jeans, the old pair leaves your home. If you get a new black dress, then an old black dress goes. You also want to buy at places you know your clothing will last a few years.

It is becoming tougher to buy quality clothing. But, it is possible. In fact, you can spend $100 and get a new wardrobe versus $300 to $1,000 for your new look.

Recently, a private study was conducted. A person bought new items from Dressbarn, spending $100 on two items. After six months, those items needed to be replaced because the fabric faded and in one case, the sweater developed a hole within the first month of wear. The person didn't wear these two items every week, but every couple of weeks.

The person then went shopping at stores like Walmart. In the same amount of time, the color faded and a few items had hem issues, where the thread unraveled. The price for those items was $20. In the same amount of time, the clothing became damaged with use, yet the less expensive clothing was more cost effective and budget friendly.

You may not be able to build a wardrobe with clothing that lasts more than six months, even if you shop at the most expensive stores. It is a fact of our consumerist society. But, you can shop with an eye towards savings and cost effective purchases.

Spending $50 on a dress that you can find for $20 somewhere else is not cost effective. It is also not a minimalist thought process. You are not being told to look frumpy, rather you are being asked to shop with savviness. Outlets, Old Navy, Walmart, and other inexpensive stores have some adorable clothing that you can look great in. Other sources like Amazon sellers with imported clothing can also help you save on your purchases.

To think like a minimalist, consider ways you can make a few outfits work for an entire week. You may feel it necessary to have new pants and shirts on every day, or you may work in an industry that allows you to wear clothes a few times before washing them again.

It may not sound clean to you, to wear pants, two or three times before washing them again. It is okay, for others it is acceptable because they know they have not sweated or had cause to truly dirty their outfit. It is your personal preference, just make certain you reduce the amount of clothing you have, buy frugally, and adapt to other minimalist ways—if you don't like compromising on clothing.

Chapter 18: Exploring Minimalism And Health

Follow these simple tips to improve your health. You will save a lot of time and a lot of money too.

Step 1: Eat well; eat simply

One of the greatest problems in the current world is that nutrition has become something complicated. It is madness, really… our great grandparents would be mortified at just how complex the concept of food has become. You have diet fads that explode onto the scene, only to be pushed out by yet another fresh diet fad.

To get the best out of nutrition, you need to keep it simple. Cut down on the processed stuff and eat lots of veggies, fruits, nuts, seeds, beans and legumes. Eat your eggs, dairy, fish & seafood and meat & poultry. If you are a vegan, you could always eliminate the animal products and enjoy your veggies, fruits and seeds.

You may still indulge in processed foods, but the idea is to do so minimally. This way, you do not have to have a bad time during birthdays, holidays and anniversaries as everyone else but you gorges on cake.

Step 2: Move your body in ways you enjoy

You do not have to embrace traditional exercises to effectively exercise. Sure, if you fancy, you could join your local gym. But you really don't have to if you don't want to. You can stack bodyweight routines on your living room floor, use free weights, perform resistance training, Etc.

Take full advantage of the local parks and hike trails. You could ride a bike too while you are at it. Trying out a new hobby is a great way to unearth new passions and better appreciate your body for the many wonderful things that it is capable of. If you have a family, why not carry out your exercises with them? Not only will it be a thousand times more fun; you will ensure that your family members raise their fitness levels and overall life quality. It's a bit like hitting two birds with one rock, really.

Here's the other thing: while the specific things you do are certainly important, they are nowhere near as important as the consistency you do them. If you can move your body for 30 minutes each day, the progress you make in just 1 year will be terrific. Not only will your physical body tell a story; you will notice that your stamina levels will improve vastly and your mental strength will grow.

Step 3: Focus on the lifestyle, not so much the goals

One of the greatest sayings is "the journey is the destination." Go through some interviews that feature rags-to-riches personalities: you will realize that while they deeply enjoy their current status, they are most excited when they talk about the harder times when they had to overcome numerous challenges and muster their willpower. Most people fail to realize this, perhaps because most people never accomplish truly great things; but the sweetest bit of success is the journey.

Even if you have A LOT of weight to shed off, do not exclusively focus on the goal in mind. Concentrate on the daily grind… focus on your repeated training routines and the work you have to put in. Focus on enjoying delicious, healthy foods and moving your body in ways that you greatly enjoy. Do these things and the added benefits of shedding weight and building lean muscle will surely come.

Step 4: Do all these things for all the right reasons

This is perhaps the most important step in this chapter, and likely the most apt piece of advice in the entire book, and here's why: you will NEVER develop any true consistency if your reasons are superficial, or they revolve around other people. The motivation will be far too fleeting and shallow; the satisfaction you gain will never really measure up to the effort you put in. If you are getting fit to impress random fellows you will bump into at the beach, come summer, you are also opening yourself up to a world of potential hurt, should there be others in better shape at the beach.

Most images and messages hugely revolve around aesthetics; it is all for the sake of improving how you look. This propaganda will really just be a waste of your time and mental/physical energy. The goal should be to eat well and improve yourself. The idea is to discover the many wonderful things that your body is capable of. Getting strong and then staying that way will ensure that you stay free of injuries and age like fine wine. Developing agility will ensure that you are able to keep doing the things that you enjoy, as well as trying out new ones.

Focus on applying all of these tips on a consistent basis and they will truly pay off.

Chapter 19: Declutter The Living Room

It is unbelievable how disorganized a living room or den can become in such a short amount of time. Here are a few tips to be sure you cover all of the areas where clutter might be taking over your living space without you realizing the problem.

You will want to begin with the same boxes for keep-toss-donate-or trash. It is easier if you wipe each of the 'keep' items while you have it in your hands. If you have children, include them in on the action. You might not mean it but play a game/trick and inform him/her if their belongings aren't out of the collection boxes in fifteen minutes; they will be gone. It might not work, but you tried! The point is to remove everything from the space that doesn't belong.

Books & Magazines

Quickly, sort through the clutter of magazines and books that have accumulated and discard, recycle, or donate the ones you have already read. Place the books on the bookshelves after you have wiped down the covers.

The secret to magazines is learning when you have enough of them. If you have a huge stack, maybe you should reconsider rejecting the renewal except for your favorite ones (not all of them)!

Consider donating the discarded magazines and books to a nursing home facility or retirement home. Some of the books might be considered for donation to local schools, libraries, or even to correctional facilities. At any rate, you need them out of your house.

Sorting the Shelves

Comb through each shelf and decide how many knickknacks you really need on one shelf. The 'dust-collectors' are so cute on the shelf in the store but can make clutter quickly. Of course, it doesn't mean you need to toss Grandma's favorite teacup. Within reason, keep the cherished ones or consider passing them on down the generation line to achieve a clean and clear atmosphere in your space.

Browse through all of the movies and DVDs. Eliminate any empty cases that don't have a use anymore. You can recycle them or donate them along with the movies you won't be viewing again. Discard any damaged or scratched movies.

Sort through all of the end tables, and remove any garbage, loose papers, or unnecessary items. Use your keep-toss-donate boxes to stay organized. Remember; don't think about the item except momentarily.

Rearrange the Book Shelves

You can make a bookcase more presentable if you remove all of the covers that are tattered and torn and place them elsewhere. You want to place focus on serenity, and you cannot do that if you are looking at the ragged edges of a book.

You can achieve an attractive backdrop by using a little bit of paint or adding some wallpaper to your space. Mix some round vases or pictures into the scenery next to a column of your nicely organized special books. Mix and match until you have a unique setting fit for a showroom.

Many organizers believe you should use one-third accessories, one-third books, and one-third empty spaces. Mix the shelves with 60% of the books placed vertically and 40% placed horizontally to create both spontaneity and balance. The point is not to make it too busy.

Take a picture in your mind or one on the phone to remind yourself of how good everything looks right now. Every three to six months, take the books down and dust the tops and spines. Flip through the pages and rotate the books to prevent any warping.

If you want to add some new dazzle to the area, consider adding some battery-operated candles to accent your newly arranged space.

Maintain the Kid's Toys

Children's toys will require some teamwork. Go back to the keep-toss-donate

boxes, and keep them handy. If your children are older, let them help with the process. If not, it might be easier to do the job—solo. Make a choice by deciding if they are toys or items the children use actively.

If they are for a younger age group, it's best to remove them from your space. Of course, you don't need to throw away the Three Bears book. However, you can place it into the bookcase instead of the toy box. (More on kids later.)

Walls - Stairs & Landings

The walls should be wiped down with warm soapy water. Don't forget to clean the baseboards. You can see dust bunnies across any room!

If you have any stairs or landings in your home, you will need to thoroughly clean each step with a whisk broom, a hand-held vacuum or a damp rag. If there are carpet sections, be sure to get along the edges thoroughly.

For all handrails and pickets; wipe each individual piece and around the bottom to remove any dirt that might have been captured.

For all spaces, use the crevice tool and brush attachment to remove the debris from the edges of the wall/baseboards.

Oil Stains on Carpet: If you have carpeted areas that have oil stains; you can use cat litter or baking soda on it to absorb the oil. Even professionals use this process.

Clean All Ceiling Fans

If you have ceiling fans, the living room is the best place to start. Since you are cleaning the house from top to bottom; it is best to pull out the vacuum cleaner hose and the broom to remove all of the cobwebs from the ceilings. Don't forget to check the fan since it will be circulating clean, fresh air. A dusty fan can ruin all of your hard work. The process only takes about fifteen minutes.

To clean the blades, this is all you need to do:

● Step 1: Tape the fan's switch for safety, so it doesn't accidentally get turned on while you clean the blades.

● Step 2: Place some old sheets or a drop cloth on the floor and remove any furniture under the fan. The blanket/drop cloth should cover a radius of approximately two that of the blades of the fan.

● Step 3: Use a spray bottle filled with water and 2 Tablespoons of distilled white vinegar. Spray the inside of an old/damaged pillowcase and place it under each fan blade.

• Step 4: Cover your head with a baseball cap.

• Step 5: Stand on a ladder to place your head above the blades.

• Step 6: Slip the pillowcase over each blade to remove the bulk of the dust.

• Step 7: Use a clean cloth to dust the lingering dust and the light fixture.

Be sure to perform these steps before you vacuum the floors.

The Heating/AC Vents

Check the heating vents, and remove any buildup of dust in each space of the home. Change the filter.

As preventive maintenance, once each month:

• Vacuum the unit with the crevice tool.

- Remove the cover and soak it in soapy water.

- Scrub it with a soft brush.

Remember to have the ductwork cleaned out about every three to five years.

Clean the Couches & Chairs

If you aren't sure, the fabric of your couch the manufacturer should have a label somewhere indiscreetly sewn into the seam of the fabric. Check underneath the cushions or the base of the furniture. You should see a label with some of the following descriptions:

- SW: Water or Solvent cleaner is safe to use.

- W: Okay to use water for cleaning.

- S: Use only solvent-based cleaners.

- X: Use Only the Vacuum for cleaning.

Once you have decided how to proceed with the type of cleaner, use this process to clean the soiled couch or chair.

● Step 1: Use a brush or white cleaning rag to groom the entire space to help remove any dried-on spots of food or other debris.

● Step 2: Sprinkle a large amount of baking soda over the entire couch. The soda will help to absorb any nasty smells and helps break up any stains lingering in the fabric.

● Wait for 20 minutes to an hour before you use the brush attachment of your vacuum cleaner to sweep away the powder.

● Step 3: Clean the sofa with the below cleaner if needed.

Cleaning Tip: Be sure to test an unnoticeable spot before you spray the entire sofa.

Chapter 20: Declutter Your Digital Life

Have you ever had a situation where your computer tells you there's no more space on the hard disc? Or where you want to take a photo, but you're out of storage space on your phone, so you frenetically go through your pictures and delete them randomly? When you can finally take a photo, the moment is gone. Since we live in a digital space, our digital clutter, junk files, and unused applications are also things that pile up if we don't take care of them. Although this clutter won't stand in your way physically, it has the same impact on your life as any other kind. However, our digital clutter is often something we put off until it can't be ignored anymore.

If you want to adopt a minimalistic lifestyle, you need to apply it to your digital life as well. Here we'll talk about all of it—from your phone and applications to photos, videos, documents, and your inbox. The main goal is to become more intentional about how you use media and technology.

Declutter your documents. Go through and delete all of the documents you no longer need. Treat your desktop the same way as your physical desktop. You wouldn't keep piles of paper on it, would you? It should be nice and clean, so keep only what you use at least on a weekly basis. While deciding what to keep and what to send to the recycle bin, avoid "just in case" syndrome. You need it or you don't. Not "just, maybe, if."

Once you've deleted everything that you don't need or use, archive and organize the files that you've decided to keep.

Make lean and simple solutions for documents that you often use. You should also find some backup solutions. This may be an external hard disc or in the cloud.

You'll notice that the majority of stuff that takes up storage space are videos and images. No matter how many of them you have, weed them. Delete all the duplicates and unnecessary pictures and videos. Keep only those you actually like and want to keep. Store them in a safe place, the cloud, or an external hard drive. Otherwise, if something happens to your computer, you will regret it and be very sad you've lost them.

When it's about photos on your phone, it's the same case. Send all of them to the computer and securely store them.

Manage the applications on your phone. All the apps you haven't used for six months or more, you can delete. If you ever need them, you can always reinstall and uninstall them again.

Clean up your social media. If you are one of those people who unintentionally scroll down the status feeds and waste time looking at a bunch of things you don't care about, it's time to do something. Unfriend and unfollow profiles and pages, leave groups you don't care about. Ask yourself: would I wish a happy birthday to this person? If yes, you should be friends on Facebook or Instagram. If not, you shouldn't have them as virtual "friends."

Deal with your inbox. It can seem like a wild, out of control beast. Unsubscribe from emails that you won't open and read. For all the email you get, try to take action immediately. Archive it, reply, do what is needed, and move it from your inbox to where it belongs. Ideally, you should reach zero in your inbox, which means that you don't have anything there. You wouldn't let your physical mail pile up in the mailbox. Treat your digital inbox the same way.

An awesome thing I like to practice every so often is that every time I notice I'm becoming too glued to my phone, I do a digital detox. I sometimes practice it for seven days, sometimes for two weeks, or even a month. The goal is to become more intentional about using media, and the benefits are numerous. Every time I notice I'm more conscious, centered, focused, and relaxed. The rules for the detox are pretty simple:

Schedule all your email activity for once a day. All the checking, answering, and whatever you have to do with email, do it at a certain time each day. The rest of the day, resist the urge to check your inbox.

Limit your social media time to half an hour a day. There's no point in mindlessly scrolling down Facebook or Instagram.

Limit all streaming to one hour daily. Here I think of YouTube, Netflix, podcasts, whatever you like to watch or listen to.

Customize notifications so they don't distract you.

Keep all the screens out of your bedroom. Your sleep will improve without the blue light from your phone and if you share a bed with a significant other, your partner will be glad too.

These are some general rules I follow each time I need to detoxify from technology and too much information. This might work for you or it might not. So I encourage you to develop your own rules for a digital diet and find out what will work best for you.

What I realized practicing this is that social media doesn't make me more connected. I was scared at first that something might go wrong if I took a break, but nothing collapsed and my relationships never suffered from taking a digital detox. I feel much happier and experience more contentment. Also, I am far more productive and focused. This all helps me create a healthy relationship with technology and use it for the highest good.

Of course, nothing's wrong with a little TV, social media, and other passive entertainment at the end of a busy day. But it's important to set a limit and maintain it.

Conclusion

There are people whose identities are attached and defined by their possessions. So when they get rid of those they feel lost. If this is you, take the time to discover who you are, regardless of what you own or lack. What's your favourite food/ animal/ song? What do you enjoy doing in your free time? What's your favourite childhood memory? What skills have you mastered? Perhaps you've always wanted to learn how to play the guitar, well now's the perfect time as you will have more time available to take care of yourself and do what you enjoy.

What would you do if you won the lottery? Chances are you would buy tons of different things and also believe you're going to be happy. Reality is that unless you were happy before winning the lottery you wont be after getting all that money. You are also very likely to lose all of it within a few years as you lack the financial education to make that money in the first place, let alone how to keep it. Happiness comes from within and it's something you need to work on daily. Don't let bad news disturb your state. Find happiness within yourself rather than looking for it on money, object or other people. Invest in yourself and love yourself.

If you are considering a conversion to the minimalist lifestyle, reflect very carefully on your reasons for doing so. You are going to embark on a journey that might change your whole life but you need a motive to keep going if you were to face a difficult time.

You can apply minimalism to almost anything but you first need to ask yourself if that's actually something you'd like to do. Maybe you like a minimalist wardrobe but you could never decorate your house in a minimal way. It's all up to you and your preferences. Minimalism is supposed to be an instrument in your life to help you have more time, space and freedom, not an obligation that you need to maintain just for the aesthetic or because it's trendy.

Minimalists in general have more time in their hands and they spend most of their time doing important things. Having quality time with your loved ones is very important but so is having a designated time to do income generating activities as well as personal development ones.

Minimalism has lately become a trend but few take the time to consider the impacts and consequences on oneself and those around us. People are rushing into minimalism and then give up as fast as they started. Enjoy the journey and let minimalism help you live a better life.

CPSIA information can be obtained
at www.ICGtesting.com
Printed in the USA
BVHW041712190121
598137BV00012BB/859

9 781989 744642